The Cause

And Cure

Of Human

Illness

Kranke Menschen
By
Arnold Ehret

The Ehret Literature Publishing Company, Inc.
P O Box 24
Dobbs Ferry, New York 10522-0024
www.arnoldehret.org

Second Edition

ISBN 1-884772-02-1

Printed in the United States of America

Acknowledgements

The translator, Prof. Dr. Ludwig Max Fischer, thanks Peter Moore for his editorial assistance; Gabriella Martinelli for her love and support; Alvin and Nita Last for their tireless commitment to preserve the Ehret heritage for our times; and finally Arnold Ehret himself for his inspiring vision, his personal dedication, and his wisdom and courage to write and live against the grain and leave humanity with a link to what is true and natural.

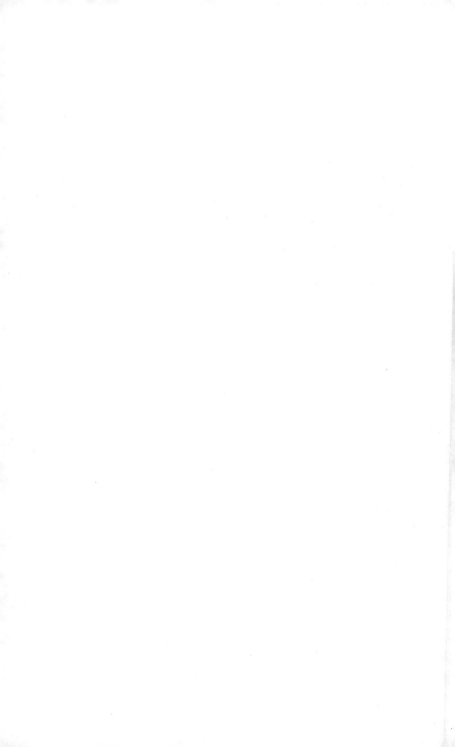

To our good friend Ludwig Max Fischer without his wonderful and difficult work this treasure could not have been published.

– Nita & Alvin

Introduction

It has been almost a hundred years since Professor Arnold Ehret wrote this book. While his other works "The Mucusless Diet Healing System" and "Rational Fasting" have withstood the test of time, staying continuously in print through many editions, "Kranke Menschen" ("The Cause and Cure of Human Illness") has remained unavailable for most of the 20th century, even in the German original. It has never been published in English.

What could an author writing shortly before the outbreak of World War I have to tell us today? We have many thousand times more the information available than he did. We have developed antibiotics, organ transplants, artificial kidneys, heart bypass operations, tranquilizers, and tens of thousands of drugs since the times of Professor Ehret, when gasoline was bought in the apothecary and the barber was also the dentist equipped mainly with a pair of pliers. Most of the sophisticated diagnostic tools, the surgical procedures and the medical technology of today were beyond the imagination of Ehret's time.

Who would question the gigantic advances of science, the results of huge laboratories, the massive body of research in innumerable journals? The medical profession, the pharmaceutical companies and the insurance industry have become massive economic institutions in every industrialized nation. Thousands of diseases have been named and classified. Research is on the way to costing billions of dollars. It seems just a matter of time and money until we solve the riddle of cancer, AIDS, Parkinsons, MS, ADD, etc. "A drug will be found" proclaim the university professors and heads of prestigious clinics almost daily in the media.

During most of the 20th century the allopathic

physician and the drugstore had almost no competition. The "quacks" and "charlatans", the homeopaths and healers relying on herbal folklore were dismissed, their organizations dismantled after the Flexnor Report in 1911. Stringent criteria for scientific evidence, empirical, analytical, double-blind, repeatable experiments exposed other approaches to health and disease as frauds punishable as criminal offenses. The naturopathic herbalist Benedict Lust, a contemporary of Professor Ehret working in New York, is said to have been jailed 27 times.

But strangely we have witnessed, during the 1980's and 1990's and continuing today, a renaissance of old fashioned nature-based approaches to health. "Alternative" and holistic healing modalities have become immensely popular again. Oriental medicine and indigenous ways of healing from around the world are drawing great interest from people from all walks of life, in spite of the fact that such treatments are not usually covered by insurance companies.

What has happened? Are we witnessing a return to an uneducated, irrational, gullible, snake-oil & witchcraft based approach to health care? Is this a sign of the decline of modern medicine?

No. The millions of suffering people defecting from Western medicine do so because they have learned from painful, direct experience that the procedures and sophisticated tests, the pills and cuts, often do not cure their ailments. They have begun to suspect that the conventional medicine might not have all the answers. The apparati may be getting bigger, along with the bills and the privileges. Medical profits are at an all time high, but the results are discouraging.

The voices of medical heretics are heard by more and more people. The books of Ivan Illich, Robert

Mendelsohn, Larry Dossey, Gabriel Cousens and others show Western medicine's accomplishments and failings in a very different light. They dare to express and explain the unthinkable and unspeakable—the recognition that Western medicine might be moving in the wrong direction. The costs of our techno-pharma-medicine bear no relation to its success in the treatment of real people. It has become itself an ideology, a potential threat to the health and economy of the industrialized nations. More people are getting sicker at earlier ages. The human body is in worse shape than ever.

We have fallen out of harmony with the forces of nature and the universe. We are losing our connections with the earthly and the divine and are creating an artificial substitute world, with our medicines and procedures that burden, irritate and weaken the body to an unsupportable and unbearable degree.

Can we take Rousseau's advice "Retour a la nature" into the 21st century? Have we truly gone forward, and can we still "go back to nature"?

Now that we have our kitchen cabinets and bathroom counters full of supplements, pills, tablets, capsules, meal replacements, slim shakes, stimulants, relaxants, antidepressants, patches and sprays, could we dare to admit that none of these expensive little bottles and gadgets will bring about the renewal of health and vitality that we seek?

Is it true that most people would prefer to suffer and even die rather than face the embarrassing possibility that true strength, health, vitality and happiness might not depend on the next super-drug? Who in our modern time can admit that health might depend on very simple, inexpensive, commonly available, well-known, ancient foods which have supported and sustained human survival and the continuity of life for millennia?

Our advanced technological ego pride will wage fierce wars against the insight and the empirical proof of a truth presented by Professor Ehret to the public a hundred years ago: Simplicity and moderation, eating mostly fruits and vegetables and a few nuts and seeds, will have a more powerful impact on the health and vitality of a person than the latest million dollar techno-medical gadget.

Western lifestyles systematically abuse the body, block its natural healing forces, separate the human being from a harmonious, vitalizing, health sustaining interaction with the pure elements of nature. We are victims of our own abuse of nature. We are driving ourselves ever deeper into serious states of degeneration and, when the inevitable decline becomes obvious, we bank our hopes for survival on some last grasp, immediate crisis, drastic intervention, emergency medical procedure.

Something has gone terribly wrong with our world-view, with our expectations, with our attitude towards the life process and its different stages, with our place in nature and our purpose and responsibilities towards the larger orders, rhythms and transformations in the cosmos. Man, the supreme manipulator, to whom the rest of creation must instantly obey, standing at the pinnacle of his evolution armed with the most advanced techno - and info-tools, is reaping the harvest of his hubris, as the ancient Greeks would have put it. This harvest of hubris includes hospitals filled with pain and disease, despair and depression, confusion and contradictory advice. This harvest of hubris includes the thousands of worthless diet fads, the thousands of new miracle substances thrown on the market and heavily advertised with great hype and promise.

But in the midst of this empty harvest of medical hubris, more and more people are taking their health back into their own hands and looking for solutions not driven by the agendas of power, profit and privilege. People are searching for affordable, effective, available healing modalities that view human suffering not as a repair job, a replace-the part-for-the-moment operation.

True healing is not about masking and suppressing symptoms. There are resources available, and caring, compassionate healing practitioners who help the person in a health crisis to empower himself and renew his vitality, often beyond most optimistic expectations. Some of the most powerful, most effective, and least expensive methods to restore a person's health are contained in the recommendations presented in this book. These recommendations are based on personal, empirical research and the results have been replicated by thousands of suffering people who overcame the most serious health challenges.

For the person who wants to live a long and healthy life, who is willing to take full responsibility for their personal well being, Professor Arnold Ehret's teachings offer real hope. For a hundred years now, these teachings have inspired individuals to achieve a better life. Every single person who has put Ehret's insights into practice has experienced profound positive changes.

There is an old saying, "Hell is preferable to the unknown." Ehret himself was aware that the majority of sufferers themselves will hang on to their pain, dismissing his teachings without ever trying them. But if it is true that a majority of people living in the hell of failing health will prefer the known, conventional pharmaceutical drugs and medical interventions to the unknown of simple diet and lifestyle change, it is equally true that growing numbers of sufferers are willing to try Ehret's radically simple approach.

Ehret's explanations for why people get sick are accessible, clear and understandable for everyone. Science for him is not an esoteric practice which invents an incomprehensible, albeit impressive, set of terms coupled with a gigantic instrumentarium. Science for Ehret is not a huge machine of projection and outward blame, trying to catch and kill an ever elusive, ever increasing "army" of microbial "enemies". Science is our responsibility to listen and harmonize with nature, and consistently live in accordance with the principles that extend and vitalize our life force as an optimal experience to be transmitted from generation to generation. Ehret took great care to phrase his insights into the causes of human illness in such a way that they make sense and have meaning for every thinking human being open to logical argumentation.

Nobody is asked to get involved in strange deprivation practices, subscribe to convoluted, abstruse theories, buy expensive supplements or meal replacements, attend high-priced seminars, weigh in weekly or draw up complex lists to be posted on the refrigerator prescribing what should and should not be eaten each breakfast, lunch and dinner. Ehret does not require complex regular diagnostic tests, medical supervision or special equipment of any kind. All that is necessary to enjoy the benefits of the Professor's time-tested teachings is to simplify your life, spend considerable less time and money on food and give his recommendation a chance for a few months.

Why then are there so few Ehretists? First, it is hard to admit that we have become addicted to eating habits which are not good for our body. Most people live on a heavily advertised and readily available diet of fast, denatured, over-processed food loaded with artificial colors, artificial flavors and chemical preservatives which extend the shelf life of the product, but actually shorten the self-life of the consumer. We eat ourselves sick for decades until the protective, inner balancing powers of our body are worn out to such a degree that illness indicates a serious deterioration process is under way. The symptoms we suffer from are in reality a benevolent physiological warning urging us to return to a more health promoting lifestyle. The war against symptoms and the mindless oppression of these warning signals in the interest of the "quick fix" is one of the most destructive, medical standard attitudes in the modern Western world. As somebody once so aptly said: "Health is built, not bought".

The second obstacle to follow the Ehret way of eating is the unfortunate "discipline" and the locked up willpower we extend toward defending our health destructive addictions to those dead, sugar- and salt-loaded poisonous food products which we use to tickle our ever less sensitive palates. The quick sugar high, the prompt, full, heavy feeling after refined cooked flour products lets us know that we are at the moment "stuffed", but that's not the same as being nourished, much less energized. In fact, our body must utilize its own stored resources of enzymes, minerals and vitamins to "neutralize" the nutritional insult. Over time such dead food attaches to our body and increasingly depletes and weakens our physical, innate defenses until we inevitably collect the harvest of empty calories in the form of disease.

A plethora of eating disorders in the majority of the population may be infinitely more dangerous to the future of our civilization than the officially recognized addictions to alcohol or illegal drugs. Our eating habits are not in harmony with the order of nature. Our digestive system transforming food intake into energy has evolved over millions of years through constant interaction with available food sources and our ability to use them. We need to eat what is good for us, has been good for us and will be good for us. If we assign an exciting taste value to a new artificial product we need to bring the manipulated taste into harmony with the life-sustaining principles of nature. Ultimately we always pay for every violent, arrogant act against nature. The Ehret way of eating guides us gently, but firmly—with flavorful, living, nourishing, great tasting food—towards regaining our connectedness with the abundance of nature. There is no need to stay addicted to nutrient-deficient food products which then cause endless worries about nutritional deficiencies in this or that newly discovered essential vitamin or enzyme. Nature provides what we need in perfect form, readily available and easily assimilable. It is the adulterations, the manipulations, the greed for profit over purity which is at the source of our pains, our allergies, our addictions. Instead of unleashing a war against "evil microbes" Arnold Ehret teaches us, first, to stop hurting ourselves every time we swallow something, and second, to watch the unimpeded healing powers of a clean and clear body move infallibly toward a vibrant, dynamic state of health and longevity. Dropping the falsely perceived obligation to self-injury while eating is the only sacrifice Ehret asks of us.

The third reason why Ehret's natural way of eating has not yet replaced the Standard American Diet (SAD) is because Ehret maintains that it is futile to search for thousands of different solutions for thousands of classified diseases when all we need to do is stop creating the problem. For Ehret there is one problem and one solution. This solution was discovered a long time ago: stop stuffing your body with substances which do not belong in there, substances which disturb the natural digestive process. It is against these substances that our body must find ways to insure normal functioning. If the body cannot somehow eliminate them, it must at least "park" or incorporate the toxic residues of unusable harmful food (or rather poison) intake. The result is an insidiously slow and silent increase of mucus in the body over decades; a very slow clogging of the villi in the colon (where 80% of our immune system activity resides); and a silt-like build up of toxins in the liver, the kidneys, and all organs of elimination. These processes cause the eventual breakdown of the most over-burdened body part or of the weakest organ due to heredi-tary imbalance. The inevitable result is a sick body mani-festing disease at a specific location, but the whole system needs to be re-balanced.

When we read about the billions of dollars spent on health-related research and applications (with ever-delayed future expectations for a possible cure), it is difficult to believe that a solution to men's modern ailments already exists. It becomes even more difficult when you know that this solution was proposed and articulated by a nutritionist, in a book written almost a hundred years ago.

Is it really heresy at the beginning of the 21st centu-ry to place our trust in following the path of nature? Is it bizarre, perverse, stupid and strange to cleanse a sick body, to purify, to remove toxins, eliminate mucus, and return to a natural lifestyle? Is it mad to trust the body's natural healing abilities, basing that trust on the empirical foundations of millions of years of survival establishing lasting harmonies between internal and external conditions?

Arnold Ehret's teachings do not require us to become rebels who feel they need to destroy before they can rebuild. Ehret's reform can be done by everyone in the pri-vacy of their own home or in any public restaurant or social gathering. Every menu and every party buffet and certainly every grocery store around the corner provides the basic ingredients. Nobody forces us to commit this slow gustatory suicide with the daily self-insult to our digestive system. Ehret shows us an easy, enjoyable way away from disease.

We do not need to convert an apple, a carrot and an almond into "applicin", "carrotol" and "almondoxin" so that the isolated "active ingredient" of the plant food source can do some good in our body. We do not need to treat the gift of the earth with a hundred artificial additives, and then rely on its enticing packaging to lure us into a purchase of dead, adulterated, processed, contaminated body burdening product. Dare to say NO to dead food. Think fresh.

Exercise your choice and eat when hungry. When sick, give your digestive system a rest. Too much is more dangerous than occasional abstinence from food. Arnold Ehret's famous fasting experiments are often misunderstood as invitations to be repeated by novice practitioners of a different way of eating. He conducted this empirical research on his own body after years of cleansing and revitalizing. He proved that for a person who has grown up on a diet considered "normal" in a Western civilization, the burden imposed on the body by excess intake of poor quality food is much more dangerous, causing many more diseases, than a temporary "scarcity" of a specific nutrient. Instead of worrying incessantly about whether we get enough of this vitamin and that mineral, we should be concerned about how the excess intake of worthless foodstuff impedes our absorption abilities and clogs up the digestive system. Deficiencies are mostly a result of excess blocking the natural processes of absorption and integration in their dynamic balances with the processes of elimination and purification. The stuffed, starving, over-stimulated sufferer does not need drastic "counter-stimulants" called drugs. Rather he needs to allow space and time for the internal elimination channels to work through the accumulated debris and unmanageable waste, to regain their effectiveness. During these times less intake means more and faster regaining of health. Minimal intervention, minimal burdening of the body with anything that requires additional energy to burn off—these have been not only the insights of Arnold Ehret, but the principles of every great physician working with nature instead of against it since at least the time of Hippocrates. Tiredness, sluggishness and many pains disappear after such fasting periods. Physical energy and mental outlook, emotional equanimity and spiritual inspiration provide exhilarating experiences for the person who has the courage to go against the grain of the conventional over-consumption imperative and experience for himself that, for a suffering body, less food almost always means more health.

Western medicine's great forté is in the dramatic, drastic crisis intervention whereby big and complex surgical procedures and powerful drugs with almost instant effects turn the tables against a life-threatening predicament of someone injured in an accident, or a stroke sufferer or a heart attack patient. Western medicine's reputation is a mystique built upon the miracle of modern technology, where heroic measures are routinely employed to remove a fast growing tumor that would otherwise be terminal. But in all this drama and crisis and emergency, we have lost the larger perspective. We have grown used to speaking of cancer and stroke victims out of context from the genesis of such diseases, ignoring the fact that 99.9% of these and all diseases stem from decades of "normal" food habits, as Ehret maintains. The successful crisis intervention is never a real solution to the problem. Inevitably, the problem will reoccur unless the original cause of the problem is addressed. In rare cases can we justify our cries for help from the doctor, nor can we blame or praise any doctor for our lost or restored health. We must return to the original role of the "doctor" (Latin for "teacher") and request the following: "Teach me to help myself in times of lost balance". Arnold Ehret does not treat patients with prescriptions, diagnoses and prognoses. Arnold Ehret teaches people to treat themselves well according to the eternal principles of balance and harmony in nature. "Natura sanat", "nature cures" was already understood in ancient times. Those who eat live, natural food in quantities agreeable to the body will not need the help of a doctor. Conversely, those who eat dead, denatured, over-processed food cannot be helped by a doctor.

The book you are about to read is an invitation coming from a truthful, sincere and original voice. Many readers, often after only a few pages, hear the message of Arnold Ehret as the somehow familiar confirmation of a long lost but reclaimable truth they have always carried within themselves. They recognize Ehret as a messenger who expresses what was hidden behind a myriad of modern confusions. They resonate with the clarity of insight and the cogent structure of his reasoning. They take heart and hope from the inspiration of such a brilliant mind, the enthusiasm of a compassionate soul and the timeless presence of a great spirit.

After the last page some may put the book aside and open the refrigerator door to finish off some leftover pieces of the sugar and starch bomb called cake they find in there. Others—and hopefully you belong to these individuals—clean out their refrigerator, reach for an apple and begin their journey to a more fruitful, healthful way of life.

Professor Dr. Ludwig Max Fischer
July 2001
Toronto, Canada

The Cause And Cure Of Human Illness

The Common Root Cause of All Diseases,
Aging and Death

by

Arnold Ehret

A fool once said
Man is born to suffer
Since then — God have mercy
It is the motto of all suffering fools.

—Mirza Schaffy

"KRANKE MENSCHEN" (Original German Title)
First Publication 1910
Ehret Publishing House, Munich

Translated by Prof. Dr. Ludwig Max Fischer

Ehret Literature Publishing Co., Inc., New York
First Publication in English

Preface

Parts of this book appeared in the year 1910 in the journal "Gesundheit" (Health), Zürich and in No 17/18 of the journal "Lebenskunst" (LifeArt), K. Lentze Publishing, Leipzig. These articles caused such an enormous interest that I felt it necessary to expand the material significantly and add important complementary insights.

This book was written for people who are seekers of truth from every source possible. May it especially serve those who are ill and inspire those who are concerned about the loss of youthfulness or worry about the symptoms of aging.

After only a year with an edition of five thousand copies the book "The Cause And Cure Of Human Illness" is already out of print, which proves the great resonance this book has found in the public. May the second edition open further vistas and paths for the truth this book stands for. With the exception of a few small changes the content remains the same.

Locarno, Fall 1912
Arnold Ehret

Preface to the 3rd edition

The many appreciative letters I have received in response to my book about "Human Illness" would already fill a volume by themselves. At every lecture I gave, so many copies were sold that it became necessary to print a third edition. In the meantime quite a few brochures and booklets about the benefits of fasting have appeared, which were written by naturopathic physicians and medical doctors. This has happened in spite of the enormous resistance to this, the most natural of all curative measures.

Most medical authorities and researchers still have not reached the level of awareness to recognize that there is actually only one disease, not a plethora of different diseases. There is only "human illness". Fasting and a natural diet are therefore beneficial for all diseases, depending on the degree of skillful application, though these measures may not help every ill person without exception.

In America, too, my book is a number one bestseller. A letter from Benedikt Lust, director and owner of the first naturopathic clinic of America in New Jersey, and contributing editor to the journal of "Naturopath and Gesundheits-Ratgeber" (Naturopath and Health Advisor), (Winter-Jungborn "Quisisana", Palm Beach, via Nuevitas, Cuba) dated July 23, 1913 confirms this. Benedikt Lust writes:

"The market is flooded with books about fasting: Dewey, Hascell, Sinclair, etc. But nobody has the depth of insight and experience you have and therefore we were delighted to receive your book. It is by far the best treatment of the subject from a practical as well as scientific point of view. I wish I had the means to acquire the rights to your new book and distribute millions of copies."

Fasting is now in danger of becoming another fad. We can only hope that this true miracle cure does not follow the pattern of hundreds of other short-lived diets, but rather will slowly and steadily gain ground in the public awareness to benefit every human being suffering from illness.

Locarno, Summer 1914
Arnold Ehret

Table of Contents

Introduction

The spirit of modern times differs from that of any other time in one regard: the plurality of perspectives regarding the basic questions of life. Neither the scholars, nor especially the scientists can find any kind of common ground. Scholars and scientists question everything, and in doing so, find everything increasingly questionable until finally the human being itself appears as a living question mark. Mauthner, in his critique of language, divulges a secret which everyone knows: all the questions of our times are answered as many times with "yes" as with "no". Everything proven is eventually disproven. This kind of sophism thoroughly permeates our sciences. By far the most bizarre set of diverging opinions and scientific controversies exist concerning the nature of human illness.

It is time to inform the general public about knowledge I have gained through experience. This knowledge is made freely available to those willing to hear it with an unbiased mind. To receive it requires being open to what is true, and a willingness to be convinced by the weight of evidence rather than by dominant public opinion.

It has been over a year since I published my experiences in the journal "Vegetarische Warte" (Vegetarian Observer), in which I described staying in a malaria-infested area of Italy with a former student of mine. With pulse rates between 45 and 52 we intentionally sought out malaria infested areas, sleeping outside and going on long, strenuous hikes.

I have offered my knowledge about absolute immunity against tropical fevers to all government offices of

Europe and America dealing with foreign and colonial affairs. I maintain—and I am ready to prove—that I am immune to cholera and will not contract it even when I eat unripe fruit. Furthermore, everyone who lives according to my dietary rules will also acquire total immunity. It is my duty and moral obligation to inform everyone about these findings, based on empirical, personal, scientific exploration, in order to help those people who seek strength and resist deterioration through disease.

In today's world there are two ways for ill people to conquer their illnesses. The first group of sufferers wants to eliminate their pain as quickly as possible. They want to discard the unpleasant experience of being a "case" to be treated. They are too busy to be sick. They are full of goals and overloaded with work, and their free time is filled with fun and entertainment. To get rid of this disturbance of illness, they start taking pills and potions, pop a myriad of medicines and remedies, and actually often achieve an improvement for awhile, enough so they can keep their head above water. But in reality their efforts prevent true healing and propel these people hopelessly toward their own inevitable downfall and eventual death. These are the facts of life for the unfortunate ones and they accept their fate.

Today's medical treatment modalities reflect a legitimate and scientific priority demanded by our society. It is a demand for the instant cure, the expectation of a scientific miracle to end disease. There is no reason to fight against allopathic medicine as long as one subscribes to this perspective. Allopathic medicine is responding to and filling a demand, and it does that more so today than ever.

Against this modern background, there is another

group of people with illnesses who are often characterized as the "stupid, backward people". In reality they are honest, intelligent people who still have a chance to survive. They pursue a more profound goal: to heal the root-cause of their disease and to thrive in health. This quest is difficult because, often, the true causes of disease are not recognized by the official, medical profession. These backward people want to heal the human being, not just subdue the symptom for a few hours, a few days or weeks. They want to fully restore the condition of the body to that which existed before the onset of their disease.

Whoever wants to walk the second path and truly heal himself must make sacrifices, take heart and muster courage. The sufferer must take complete responsibility, and become his own physician and therapist. The sufferer may seek council but only as inspiration and general guidance, for the real work of healing must be accomplished by himself alone. The purpose of this book is to give the person who does his own healing work a sense of direction.

Between the two poles described here, there is a third way: naturopathic medicine. But naturopathy is in a precarious position these days. On the one hand, naturopathy wants to heal the person without masking the disease, which is positive for the healing process. But naturopathic medicine often leaves the root of the illness, namely "comfort food", untouched. Whoever wants to be healed in a natural way must be willing to live in accordance with those laws which nature provides for all living creatures. These natural laws are simple, immutable and knowable. They include regular fasting, especially when ill. Nature's laws prohibit eating anything "artificial", that is to say processed and cooked foods. Specifically nature would have us regularly eat fruit and other plants. I will not deny that naturopathic medicine can support the effect of fasting through the skillful use of fresh air and water (baths). But until naturopathy fully embraces diet as cause or cure of human illness, it will remain in its precarious position.

How are we supposed to fast then? Which foods are we to eat and to avoid? This book will answer these questions. These answers are given as general guidelines and are not a substitute for concrete and individualized medical procedures determined by a qualified health practitioner on a case by case basis.

My readers have found great benefits from the information and the philosophy of healing I have espoused in earlier articles. That body of work will be enriched even more by this expanded version. Yet official medical doctrine ignores my work or dismisses it as the utopian vision of a layman. Such medieval orthodox rigidity actually disqualifies itself. When did true science, the natural sciences and technological progress, ever care whether its major explorers and inventors were "professionals" or "laymen"? Did the professional establishment not ridicule Franklin and Galvani, Edison and Zeppelin, only to eventually recognize and respect the scientific breakthroughs of these laymen geniuses? Students in medical school may occasionally hear about the benefits of a Priessnitz cold-water wrap, but they are never told that Priessnitz was a layman.

I neither believe in the completely hostile invalidation of allopathic medicine by the practitioners of naturopathic medicine, nor do I advocate any of the modern forms of quackery. I must state clearly here that many charlatans "work" in the name of "nature". My position and my evidence stand completely on their own.

I
The Common Root Cause of All Diseases

"You are a true benefactor of mankind!
I would be happy for all human beings,
If they lived in accordance with
your purely true principles."
—Heinrich Knote, Singer

All stages in the development of medicine, including the healing practices of ancient cultures, have viewed illness as an external force penetrating into the human being. These negative, evil influences disturb the normal lifestyle of the person and then, through an irreversible, irrefutable and non-negotiable progression, harm and finally kill the human being. This basic notion of an evil demon invading the healthy human has continued unchanged, even in modern medicine, irrespective of the latter's claims to "scientific" superiority. This is especially evidenced in the most advanced form of scientific medicine as it searches frantically for a new virus, new bacteria, new parasites, every day in every laboratory, eager to "catch" and identify another harmful "secret, undercover, invasive agent". From a philosophical point of view the medieval superstitions and the modern cult of microbes are the same. Then it was the "evil spirit", the "devil"; now it is a tiny devil, a literally microscopic devil, whose existence can be scientifically proven.

Now an additional term comes into play: genetic predisposition! A wonderful term. But nobody has told us what it truly means. All experiments with animals are questionable because the produced symptoms occur only with injections directly into the blood, but never through oral ingestion.

There is some truth to the idea of the external influence, i.e. that problems "come from the outside". However, this doesn't happen through the intervention of a vicious enemy attacking us. Rather, this occurs in the sense that all illnesses, including the inherited diseases, stem from biologically wrong, unnatural food, and from every gram of excess food intake. The exceptions are rare, e.g. lack of hygiene.

My first major point is that every illness, without exception, is an attempt by the body to eliminate mucus and, in advanced stages, pus (disintegrated blood). Every healthy organism of course must contain a certain amount of naturally occurring mucus, called lymph, the fatty mucus-like substance of the colon. Every medical expert dealing with cathartic problems, from a harmless runny nose to pneumonia and tuberculosis, will attest to this fact. But we are examining here a very unnatural and unhealthy mucus condition which is epidemic in modern society. The body's attempt to eliminate excess mucus is not always obvious in diseases of the ears, eyes, skin diseases, stomach problems, heart trouble, rheumatism, arthritis, etc., not to mention in mental disturbances. And yet excess mucus is the main cause of the problem. Mucus, which can no longer be eliminated through natural means, enters the blood and reappears at a location where the blood circulation is reduced (perhaps because of a strong chill) as a heat symptom, an inflammation, a pain, or maybe a fever produced by the body.

If you put a sick person on a mucusless diet, say

fruit, or even just water or lemonade, the energy usually used for digestion (and now free for the first time in decades) will immediately attack and try to dissolve the hardened masses of mucus that have accumulated in the body since childhood. And what is the result? With absolute certainty this mucus will manifest itself in the urine and feces. I call these hardened masses of mucus, present at the center of every pathological abnormality, the common root cause of every illness. If the disease is in an advanced stage, to the degree that there are pathological tissue changes deep inside the body, you will also see the elimination of pus. As soon as the mucus-forming artificial food, like fat meat, bread, potatoes, pasta, rice, milk, etc. are discontinued, the bloodstream will attack mucus and pus and will eliminate both through the urine. In people with a high degree of mucus the body will use each and every body opening and elimination channel to rid itself of the poisons.

If you cook potatoes, flour, rice, or meat long enough you will end up with a gelatin-like, thick mucus substance. It looks very much like the glue that bookbinders and woodworkers use as adhesives. This mucus-like substance soon turns acidic, starts to ferment, and becomes the breeding ground for fungi, mold, and bacteria. In the digestive process, which is, chemically speaking, nothing but a kind of cooking and brewing process, this mucus—this glue—is separated out, because blood can only absorb the glucose which has been extracted from the carbohydrates. The remaining byproduct, the mucus or glue, is an alien substance for the body, which must be eliminated completely from the earliest stage of life on.

Now it becomes clear that, in the course of a lifetime, the digestive tract and the colon are increasingly clogged up with mucus. This glue-like substance, the residue of plant and animal material, continues to ferment, and finally clogs up the arteries and affects the blood's ability to regenerate the whole system.

If, on the other hand, you cook figs, dates, or grapes long enough, until they become a thick paste, you will observe that this substance neither ferments nor forms mucus. It is therefore not called mucus by anybody, but is known by the name "syrup". Glucose, the body's most important building material, is sticky, too, but the body uses it as prime fuel without leaving any residue. Instead, it leaves behind traces of cellulose, which are not sticky, do not ferment, and are eliminated quickly. The concentrated sugar of fruit is even used to preserve because of its ability to prevent fermentation.

Every person, healthy and ill, secretes sticky mucus on the tongue as soon as he reduces his intake of food, or "fasts". The same process occurs on the stomach lining, which is an exact mirror of the tongue. You can see this mucus in the first bowel movement after a fast.

Of course my mucus theory will stir up great controversies in scientific circles, as do all discoveries originating from laymen. Therefore I will explain my theory in more detail to avoid misunderstandings.

I am not saying that mucus is always and exclusively the cause of all diseases, but I do maintain that mucus is the common basic factor of all diseases. There can be many other causes of disease and I do not deny them, but mucus will be involved in each and every case. There is evidence for mucus from childhood on, even in a seemingly healthy organism. Mucus is the main and common factor in every illness, the main substance and indicator next to uric acid, metabolic toxins, carbonic acid, etc. Residues of metabolic waste products originating from animal and plant material form a plaque in the stomach and the colon due to their glue-like, sticky characteristics. This plaque clogs up the digestive tube and is eventually carried through the bloodstream (leukocytes) into every circulatory system of the body, especially the large blood vessels. It causes the clogging of the organs of the lungs, the heart and the kidneys. Whoever does not understand that a thirty foot long tube, the digestive tract, will inevitably collect impurities and residues in its inner linings, even with the strongest digestion, cannot be helped.

My observations can be repeated and documented as an objective reality. They are demonstrable for every person through scientific experiment. They do not grow out of the overactive fantasy of a layman. I recommend to doubting medical doctors and researchers the test of the actual scientific experiment, which alone can reliably verify my theory. A scientific experiment is a question to nature and is the foundation of all natural sciences. Scientific experimentation provides us with unshakable truths regardless of the person formulating the hypothesis. Additionally, I recommend to those with the courage to prove the validity of my theories, that they report the results of the experiments I am describing in this book as part of their own experience. They will receive the same answer from nature (i.e. from their own body) that I received, provided that they are in a state of health as I define it, because exact results, precise responses, are only possible from a pure, healthy, mucus-free organism.

After almost two years of living on fruit only, with intermittent fasting periods, I attained a state of health hardly imaginable in today's world. For example, I was able to conduct experiments such as I described in my article: "A 49 Day Fasting Experiment" (published in "Vegetarische Warte" (Vegetarian Observer) 1909/10), with the following results:

When I made a cut in my forearm with a knife, there was no bleeding, because the blood coagulated immediately. The wound closed instantly—no inflammation, no pain, no mucus and no pus. In three days the wound was totally healed and the scab had fallen off. Later I repeated the experiment after eating vegetarian food including mucus-forming carbohydrates, but without eggs or milk. The result was that the wound bled a little; I had some pain and some pus oozed out of the wound. There was some inflammation and it took quite a while for the wound to heal. Some time later I conducted the same experiment while on a diet including meat and moderate alcohol. The result was an extended period of bleeding. The blood was light, red and thin, and there was inflammation, pain, and several days of pus. The wound only healed after two days of fasting.

I offered to repeat these experiments to the Prussian ministry of war, but without avail. Why did the wounds of the Japanese heal much faster and better during the Russian-Japanese war than the wounds of the "meat and vodka" Russians? Why has nobody thought for two thousand years about the fact that neither the opening of veins nor the drinking of the hemlock cup could kill Seneca after he had abstained from meat and fasted in his prison cell?

Seneca is supposed to have lived previously only from fruit and water.

   In the final analysis every disease is a clogging of the tiniest blood vessels, the capillaries, with mucus. If the pipes of a city's water supply have dirty water pumped through them because of clogged filters, nobody would think of cleaning these pipes without stopping the flow of dirty water during the repair work. More importantly, wise people would immediately direct their attention to the reservoir, the distribution center, and the faulty filters and malfunctioning pump. But these can only be fixed when the dirty water stops running. "I am thy Lord, thy healer" translates in our time as: 'Only nature heals, purifies, and de-clogs infallibly and totally—but only if you stop supplying your body with mucus-forming food'. Every physiological machine, whether human or animal, purifies itself instantly and automatically, dissolving the mucus in the clogged pipes as soon as the intake of solid food stops. During a fast, even the healthiest person will eliminate mucus, which can be detected in the urine if collected in a glass and allowed to cool. Whoever denies, ignores or suppresses this fact because it is inconvenient or not "scientific" enough, carries the responsibility of covering up the discovery of the main cause of every disease, but more so, inflicts the worst injury on himself.

   I am revealing here the true cause of tuberculosis. Does anyone still believe that the enormous amount of mucus eliminated by a TB sufferer actually comes from the lungs only? Actually, because tuberculosis patients are fed a mucus-rich diet (porridge, milk, and fat meat), mucus continues to build up until the lungs start to disintegrate and "bacteria" grow, causing further deterioration. Here the mystery of bacteria becomes quite clear. The accumulation of mucus causes a clogging of the blood vessels, which then leads to a fermentation process of these mucus-rich substances, these residues of dead cooked food. They can no longer be eliminated and begin to "spoil" in the living body, resulting in puss-filled boils, cancer, tuberculosis, syphilis, lupus, etc. It is well known that meat, cheese, and other organic matter spoil while fermenting, growing bacteria as they decay. This is why these bacteria are only detectable in more advanced stages of the disease. They are not the cause, but rather the symptom of the disease. They do accelerate the disease process, however, because the toxins produced by the growing bacteria facilitate the further deterioration of the body's organs—the lung, for example.

Doubters of this theory point out that bacteria invade an organism from the outside, as in a "contagious" disease. But here the exception proves the rule: in this case, the accumulated mucus within the organism provides a fertile ground for bacterial activity.

If it is true that bacteria invade an organism from the outside, as in a "contagious" disease, this is because the accumulated mucus within the organism provides a fertile ground for their activity, which is called "genetic predisposition".

I have lived several times in my life—once for a period of two years—on a diet without mucus, e.g. on fruit only. I do not need a handkerchief anymore and have rarely any use for this product of culture. Has anyone ever seen an animal living in the wild having to blow its nose? A young medical doctor and naturopath disagrees with my view that

the nose of a healthy animal or of a truly healthy person
should not secrete any mucus. He considers the mucus-free
nose an abnormality. Obviously he has never examined the
nose of a wild animal, or of pets for that matter. The careful
observer finds no mucus at all there, but a certain moistness,
the dew of the cool air which has the meaningful purpose to
filter dust from the in-flowing air. A mucus-free nose is not
at all a disease symptom. A mucus-free nose occurs only
when there is no intake of any mucus for awhile. I have
observed the same phenomenon with all my patients who,
by the way, felt their best when there was no mucus in their nose.

My chronic nephritis, which was considered terminal, was not only completely healed, but I am in a state of
health and energy which by far surpasses that of my teenage
years. Show me a European who is terminally ill at the age
of 31, and who runs over two hours and hikes 56 hours without interruption eight years later.

Thus my "Mucus Theory", based on repeated experiments, proposes the first thorough, universal causality of
all illnesses. Even though naturopathic doctors usually suspect blood diseases, and in particular Dr. Lahmann discusses the "dietary blood disintegration" as a basic cause for all
illnesses, this viewpoint has proven insufficient in practice.
The reason for the failure of this therapy was that, although
the diet excluded meat, it included bread, gruel, milk,
butter, eggs, cheese, and pies, and thereby, especially with
the inclusion of starch flour, introduced high amounts of
mucus into the patient.

These same factors contribute to sickness in vegetarians, whose diets are otherwise to be highly praised. I can
attest to this from personal experience, as I was, for several

years, a mucus glutton myself. If most of today's vegetarians do not find their way back to natural food and fruit-diets, or advance to mucus-free diets and learn portion control soon, there is a danger that the vegetarian movement will become a fad of the past. This is not because the concept of excluding meat from one's diet is poor, but mainly because the healing success of common vegetarian diets is so poor. The good news is that a small number of fruit-eaters is regularly taking first place in competitive foot marches and other disciplines, but conventional medicine does not acknowledge their diet as the reason for their successes. More commonly however, one finds representatives of the vegetarian movement trying to prove that humans need various types of cooked food, because they cannot bring themselves to acknowledge the foundation of the fruit-diet as a remedy.

One objective of the vegetarians' propaganda is to prove that man is not naturally carnivorous, and that meat is "unnatural". Of course critics counter—justly—that eating meat is as "natural" as eating cabbage, bread, milk, and cheese. More than a decade ago, Professor v. Bunge labeled vegetarians as inconsequential, and he is right. In scientific centers led by vegetarians, the protein and nutrient value of vegetarian meals was evaluated and misleadingly compared to the nutrient value of meat. Such a debate is beside the point. Vegetarians seem to have forgotten the famous principle of healing, which is: "The more you feed a sick person, the more you harm him." (Hippocrates, an eminent dietician and the greatest physician, father of the medical profession).

Up to now I have not been talking about fasting as a

lifestyle—not in the sense of vegetarian propaganda, but solely as a form of healing. The mucus-free diet as a means of healing conforms to Hippocrates' view of "not-feeding", i.e. not further burdening the body, but rather facilitating excretion.

Theoretically, at an earlier time in the evolution of the species, people surely lived off fruit only. Biologically, we can certainly still do that. Perhaps for some their "common sense" cannot be persuaded, without proof, that people lived from fruit only, before they became hunters. But I will go so far as to declare that human beings once lived in perfect health, beauty and unimagined strength, without pain and distress, just as it is written in the Bible. Only fruit, the sole mucus-free nourishment, is natural. Everything prepared and supposedly improved by people causes harm.

This argument concerning fruit is scientifically defensible. An apple or a banana contains everything needed to meet human dietary requirements. There are said to be old people with enormous energies who never ate anything but bananas their entire lives. The human body is perfected enough to live off one fruit only, at least for a long period of time. One should not dismiss a simple truth, preached by nature, just because cultural norms don't allow for it. It is true that, initially, a fruit-only diet always leads to sickness, but that is because the body goes through a cleansing process.

Had I not proven it by doing it, no one would have believed my assertion that during 14 months one can live 126 days—49 in a row—without food. Even now, no one understands the implications of this truth, even though I have presented empirical proof. Up to now I have taught that fruit is the most natural remedy.

The fundamental truth of this most natural way of healing is not affected by such questions as whether Eskimos, or any other people, could live this way. It doesn't matter that I myself do not absolutely live this way. What matters is the truth of healing. We will see whether my assumptions are correct when Europe is struck by the next epidemic of an infectious disease.

I want to discuss here the reasons why people are not inclined to believe the self-evident. If someone had suggested making a phone call to Paris from Berlin during the 18th century, he would have been laughed out of town and dismissed out of hand, because the knowledge of how to do that did not exist at that time. In a similar fashion, a natural foods diet is dismissed because, as civilized people, we are not used to it and, moreover, we find it difficult to even practice living a natural life. Some opponents fear a drop in the price of artificial food products, while others fear an invalidation of current nutritional science and a social devaluation of physicians. On this last point, let me be clear: As there is a need for constant monitoring and instruction regarding fasting-cures and fruit-cures, there should be an increasing number of physicians caring for a smaller number of patients, all of whom are very willing to pay more to get healed. This posits a bright future for doctors.

Most fasting experiments fail for one simple reason: People are not aware that the beginning of the mucus-free diet causes an excretion of old mucus until the patient is absolutely pure and healthy. This is a cleansing process and causes a transitional phase of sickness in an otherwise healthy person on his way to a higher level of health.

Unfortunately, because only a few vegetarians have ever personally experienced this higher level of health, the majority of vegetarians dismiss it as unobtainable. However, as chronicled in the "Vegetarische Warte" (Vegetarian Observer), my 49 day fasting experiment, preceded by a fruit-only diet, proved that the big objection of "mal-nourishment" is unfounded in regards to fasting. Irrespective of some unhygienic side effects, my general condition only improved due to the radical excretion of mucus from my body. Another good outcome of that fasting experiment was that I received countless recognitions from people in highly educated circles.

Meanwhile, the majority of vegetarians "slimes" on. Vegetarian representatives of both sexes are undifferentiated from "Munich Beer-bellies", a result of cramming in all that "mucus-food" on a daily basis. Compared to this, indicted poisons like meat, alcohol, coffee, and tobacco are relatively harmless, consumed in small amounts. Are there not thousands of people, living to advanced age, who are habitual smokers with a fondness for alcoholic beverages? They are just small eaters! This is the solution! Even these habitual toxins are less harmful than stuffing oneself regularly with good old "comfort" foods. As professor Sylvester Graham puts it: "A drunkard can get old, a glutton never."

I will present some explanations here to prevent misunderstandings among teetotalers and vegetarians. Meat is not a food. Rather, it is a stimulus that putrefies in the stomach. This putrefaction does not start in the stomach, however, but immediately after the slaughter of the animal. Graham has proved this for living humans, and I add to this fact that meat works as a stimulant through the toxins of

putrefaction, and is therefore perceived as an energy pro-
viding food. I do not believe that anybody can find chemical-physiological evidence that a putrefying protein-molecule gets transformed in the stomach to be revived in a person's muscle as available energy. Similar to alcohol and
other stimulants, meat initially appears to give strength and
energy until the whole organism is contaminated by it and
inevitably breaks down.

The basic evil of all non-vegetarian diets is the over-
consumption of meat, which leads to other evils, such as the
craving for alcohol. Eating a fruit-only diet avoids the craving for alcohol, while carnivores constantly have to fight the
lust for it, because meat calls the demon "thirst" into the
great plan of life. Evidently alcohol serves as some kind of
counter-toxin for meat. City-gourmets, primarily living off
meat, need wine, coffee, and tobacco as a partial counter-
toxin for their meat poisoning. It is a ironic matter of fact
that one's physical condition after eating an opulent dinner
will be better if the meal is consumed with small doses of
such toxic stimulants than without them.

I absolutely declare war against meat and alcohol;
eating fruit and generally eating little vigorously counter-
acts the consumption of meat and alcohol. Nevertheless,
there is great irony in the fact that people who consume both
meat and alcohol, but in small portions, are in a better position by far than vegetarians who eat too much.

The American Fletcher proves this fact through his
enormous healing successes. My experiments explain his
secret by revealing that people are most efficient and
healthy when eating as little as possible. Is it not true that
the oldest people are usually poor and therefore used to eat-

ing little for obvious reasons? Is it not true that the greatest discoverers and inventors stem from poor families and therefore ate little? Is it not true that the greatest people in human history, the prophets, founders of religions, etc. were ascetics? Why is it called culture when people living in Berlin opulently stuff themselves three times a day? Why is it called social progress when every blue-collar worker eats five meals a day and pumps his body full of beer in the evenings? Feasting, considered to be harmless, proper, moral and aesthetic up to now, is not only immoral, but is the cause of more disease than everything else, even for teetotalers and vegetarians. Given that a diseased organism best regenerates without food, it is only logical that a healthy one needs only little nourishment for health, strength and endurance.

All the holy miracles at sacred places can be ascribed to asceticism, and are rare nowadays because the prayers are no longer accompanied by fasting. There are no miracles anymore because there are no saints—people who have been sanctified and healed by fasting and asceticism. The saints were self-radiant. Speaking in modern terms, they were "mediums" or "psychics", not because of a "special grace", but because their asceticism led them to a physiologically "godlike" health.

I will mention here that I myself produced visible, electrical radiances, merely by external and internal supply of sun-power (sunbaths and food out of the "sun-kitchen", i.e. fruit). The whole world is now arguing about these phenomena and tries to explain them. The solution lies right at the center of the experiment, which anyone can repeat who has the guts to do so, as with any rigorous scientific experiment. But it is easier to write books, talk about it, pray, or view me as an exception to the norm. My experience may be the exception, but only because of the courage and consciousness I bring to it. Physiologically all human beings are equal, and he who cannot moderate himself should learn it from me, if he chooses to be a true explorer. When a person eats little and is healthy, he can digest and eliminate the most absurd food, including meat and mucus. A person becomes even more perfect and pure when eating only fruit, of which he needs very little, because fruit is the quintessential nourishment.

People of today will not and cannot accept this eternal truth dictated by natural law. They are even afraid of it, because their bodies are built of food that has been cooked to death, and they are accustomed to this. Yet their dead body cells are eliminated the moment they take a sun-bath, fast or ingest the living cells of fruit. This cure has to be done with a great deal of caution. Medicine has tried to prolong human life from cell-breakdowns for as long as possible only to let people die even faster in case of diseases when a quick death seems better than long suffering. Vegetarians cannot deny that consumers of meat and alcohol are highly effective, apparently healthy, and survive into old age, provided that such people eat little and do not get over-nourished. The meat diet contains relatively little "mucus" compared to the "slimy" vegetarian diet, which mainly consists of starch-flour, especially the highly praised vegetarian dinners with their many courses every day.

I haven't bothered with eating at prescribed times during the day for many years now. I eat only when I have an appetite and then I eat only a little, to prevent harmful effects in case I ingest food that is not absolutely healthy. The art of remaining healthy does not so much take into account the "what" we ingest but the "how much" food and beverages we take in. What is important is self-control and self-restraint. I personally consider it a bad example to advocate vegetarianism and abstinence, pretending to a pioneer of a global mission, only not to "walk one's talk" in the end. I want to dissociate my work from fanatic movements of any kind.

If it is possible to heal the most serious diseases with fasting —which is proven— and, if done right, even get stronger through this lifestyle, it follows then that fruit, which is reliably the food richest in energy, will bestow even greater health and strength.

Allopathic medicine admits that the sick organism has to excrete something, but thus far has mainly worked on the hypothesis of irritants, or counter-toxins. It often prescribes an alcohol- and meat-free diet, but ignores the real natural forces of the healing process—namely, a decrease in food, fasting and especially the fruit diet.

Alcohol is particularly viewed as a major culprit and made the scapegoat for almost every illness, because some squalid people, consuming enormous quantities of it, fall into a delirium. But just force a drunkard to stay on an all-fruit diet for a few days, and I assure you he will not find any pleasure in the best booze. Here the dangers of our cultural eating norms become obvious. Everything taken to excess, from beefsteak to supposedly harmless porridge, creates a craving for proscribed substances, like alcohol, tea, or tobacco, as an antidote, or counter-toxin. Why? The reason is that eating extensively makes a person indolent and only those irritants can get the person going again. Thus the true main reason for the increase in alcohol consumption is seen to be this over-nourishment with food, especially with meat. Alcohol, and particularly beer, acts instantly as an irritant but is, in the long run, less harmful to health than the chronic poisoning of the whole digestive tract with mucus-rich food.

Given that our bodies have accumulated masses of mucus since childhood, which now is causal to a process of deterioration in the body (which in places is evidenced as infected body-tissue, i.e. a symptom for disease), my question now is, which of the following strategies seems more reasonable? Does it make sense to force these masses of accumulated mucus out of the body by sweating, baths, artificially induced fevers (Kneipp-cures), massages, sports, etc., at the expense of vitality (mainly of the heart) and longevity? Or would it make more sense and be more effective to just stop the ingestion of mucus? The answer is obvious. If mucus producing foods and over-nourishment really are the main root causes for all illnesses without exception (a theory I can prove with my own body), then there is only one really natural remedy—fasting and an all-fruit-diet.

The mucusless diet is properly viewed as a significant step on the path to natural healing. It is well known that every animal fasts at the slightest sign of sickness, which only proves my point. Normally animals only munch as much as is necessary for them and, typically, they fast till they are healthy. If our pets have lost this instinct for the right time and the right amount of chow, it is due to the ignorance of our civilization and to the people who over-feed them in times of sickness. And if it is bad for our pets, it's worse for our people. In our misguided society, the poor sick person is not allowed to eat small or no portions for more than one or two days "for their own good", so as to not become "weakened". People are pressured to eat with the best intentions and the worst results.

Physicians who pay attention to results have described fasting as "a miraculous cure", a "cure for the incurable", a "cure of all cures", etc. Unfortunately, some charlatans, lacking the necessary basic knowledge, have brought discredit on this infallible, but hazardous cure. I hold the world-record for fasting, 49 days, (see "Vegetarische Warte" (Vegetarian Observer) 1909, Vols. 19, 20, 22; 1910, Vols. 1 and 2) and I know the rigors and rewards of this miracle cure intimately. Through my research, I have combined the basic cure of fasting with a systematically and individually adjusted fruit-diet (mucus-free diet), making it surprisingly easy and absolutely risk free. We now can reliably cure diseases that traditional medicine deems incurable. Based on my knowledge about mucus being the root cause and main factor of all illnesses, symptoms of aging, obesity, loss of hair, wrinkles, weakness of nerves and memory, etc., I envision a new age of innovative cures and biological medicine.

Hippocrates long ago realized the essence of all illness. More recently, Prof. Dr. Jaeger termed the common symptom as "malodorousness" but did not identify the source of this "bad smell". Dr. Lahmann and other advocates of the physical-dietary movement, particularly Dr. Kuhne, have searched for "common alien substances" to shed light on human disease. None, however, has been able to scientifically, through experiment, prove that the main cause for disease is the mucus in our artificially altered foods. This mucus, which burdens our organism from early childhood on, can even threaten the viability of the human organism. Beyond a certain threshold, the mucus in the body can enter a state of fermentation, building up pathological metastasis in which the body tissue starts to fester and deteriorate. Occasional colds or high temperatures activate this mucus, and in trying to leave the body, it causes symptoms of abnormal functioning, which up to now have been incorrectly identified as the illness itself. Now, for the first time, we are able to define predisposition. The more mucus is accumulated from childhood on through contaminated mother's milk or supplements, and the less mucus is metabolized and excreted by the responsible organs, the higher is the probability (predisposition) to catch a cold, develop fevers, feel cold, host parasites, fall ill or age prematurely.

This knowledge most probably lifts the veil off the secret of white blood cells. I think that our understanding here, as in many other fields of medical research, may be incomplete. Bacteria invade the white blood cells rather than the other way round, because those cells consist mainly of the perpetually indicted mucus. Outside of the organism there are millions of bacteria cultivated on exactly this mucus. They grow on potatoes, bouillon, gelatin—in a word, on slime, a nitrogenous herbal and animal substance, consisting of alkaloid reacting fluids, which contains granulated cells similar in appearance to white blood cells. Maybe an absolutely healthy mucous membrane is not supposed to be white and slimy at all, but clear and red, like the mucous membranes of normal healthy animals. Maybe the "death slime" is the true reason for the paleness of the white race! Paleface! Deathlike pallor!

This "mucus-theory", proven by experimentation, wrestles the demonic mask from the ghost of illness. Those who believe me have an opportunity not only to heal themselves, but have—for the first time ever—the opportunity to prevent sickness forever, to make it impossible. Even the dream of everlasting youth and beauty can come true here.

The mammal organism, especially the human organism, is, technically speaking, a complex pipe-system of blood vessels driven by the air of the lungs, with the blood-fluid constantly moving and being regulated by the heart as a valve. Every breath causes the splitting up of air into oxygen and nitrogen in the lungs. This constantly activates the blood, and the human body can work properly for an incredibly long time without tiring. What is completely left out of this mechanistic description is the issue of the transcendental, metaphysical life-force, the existence of which is contested by our stubbornly materialistic way of thinking.

My argument here is simple and basic: If we do not slow our engine down by excessive eating, it will work better. I do not want to listen to ignorant and uninformed excuses anymore—people talking about their "daily necessity and natural urge to eat a lot"—before those people have experienced how easy and long one can work or walk without tiring in a lifestyle that includes fasting and fruit-diet.

Getting tired is the result of three factors. The first reason for fatigue is a reduction in strength due to excessive digestion. Second is the congestion of blood vessels, because they are heated up, which causes their dilation. And finally the "self-poisoning" and "rebound-poisoning" caused by mucus-excretion due to activity. Air is not only the best and quintessential operating-substance for the human body; it is also the basic element for build-up, repair, replacement and perhaps also the source of nitrogen for the animal organism. At least there is no proof to the contrary. There have reportedly been weight gains of a certain kind of caterpillar due to air only.

II
Ways to Eliminate the Common
Root Cause of All Diseases and
Prevention of Their Reoccurrence

After presenting to my readers the horrors of disease in the previous chapter, it seems only fair now to show them ways and means to successfully fight the biggest health-enemy—mucus-poisoning.

I have already stated that individual treatment is necessary for the sick. I have been able to intervene in a helping and healing manner in numerous difficult cases, either with oral or written advice. I now want to present three paths towards health.

1. The shortest and safest path to health is fasting. It makes the enemy's life in our body unlivable, forces him to flee and he turns away in fear from us, the fasters. Healthy people can undergo a fasting-cure without any difficulties. Of course they have to fast reasonably and must bear the responsibility for not causing dangerous overexertion by trying to do physical or mental activities that would tax their resources even on a normal diet. I want to mention a security measure here, which has to be used for all fasting-cures; at the beginning of fasting the intestinal tract should be fully emptied with the use of a laxative enema, or something similar. It seems logical that the fasting person should not be additionally bothered by gases and disintegrating substances of the feces that are still in the intestines. The excretion of mucus occupies the person enough.

Those who do not dare to fast for a longer period of time should try short fasting. Even 36 hours of fasting once or twice a week has very positive effects over time. One is advised to start off by omitting dinner and doing an enema instead. Nothing is to be ingested till 36 hours later, and for that breakfast only fruit is taken. Eating fruit is necessary after each fasting period, because the fruit-juices activate the loosened masses of mucus. For sick and elderly people there has to be medical supervision. A special warning to people who regularly consume meat in their diets: Do not start right away with fasting and fruit-diet. A strictly individualized intermediate diet, instructed and supervised by a professional, is absolutely necessary. Otherwise, the abrupt change can be dangerous.

To reach the goal faster, the method discussed above is to be extended. For example, three days of fasting followed by several days of post-fast fruit diet only. This means eating nothing at all for three days (only sipping lemonade when needed), beginning with vegetables, salad or fruit on the fourth day, and taking an enema on the evening of the fourth day. Healthy people, and especially those whose job permits them to rest during the difficult times of mucus-excretion and mood fluctuations, can extend the fasting for weeks. I must stress again that these fasting suggestions are valid only for relatively healthy people who want to experience first-hand the mental and physical regeneration of fasting. Sick people are not to simply follow these common rules suggested above: they must be treated individually.

No one should be discouraged by the unattractive appearance or the loss of body weight that fasting brings. The body fasts itself healthy, despite the miserable complexion, and soon the cheeks are going to be fresh and rosy again and the weight, too, will return to normal soon after fasting. After fasting, the body reacts to every single gram of food. People who fast abstemiously will often present a fine, spiritual facial expression. Pope Leo XIII, a great faster and sage, is said to have had a clear and almost lucent complexion.

One point should be mentioned here again, as the success of fasting depends heavily on this point. It is important that the fasting person not become discouraged and depressed. Some will find that tranquility facilitates their unpleasant moments, while others prefer extensive activity, especially simple motor tasks.

After freeing the body from slime and mucus, the revitalized healthy person's duty is to keep this state sacred and maintain it in life through right nutrition.

2. People who can't fast due to health issues, like advanced lung or heart disease, should at least make sure not to pile up even more mucus in their body. They should abstain from markedly mucus-building substances, especially food prepared from flour (esp. cake), rice and potato dishes, cooked milk, cheese, meat, and so on. Cottage cheese, soured milk, and yogurt do not produce as much slime, because they work as laxatives at the same time. Those who cannot abstain from bread should eat it toasted only. The process of toasting decreases the harm, because mucus-substances get partly destroyed. Eating toasted bread has yet another advantage; one does not eat as much of it, and the necessary chewing movements bring about the tiring even of the greediest palate. Those who cannot easily chew the toasted bread due to dental problems should suck on the bread until it disintegrates in the mouth. This is an outstanding method to regain lost strength. Potatoes, if con-

sumed at all, are taken roasted only.

Again I want to advise sick people to consult a professional for guidance. Every single step in the direction of a mucus-free or low-mucus diet is different according to illness and individual condition. The correct and professionally supervised transition diet is extremely important and can't be over-stated. It is not the sick person or his relatives who decides about the course of the diet, but only the professional dietician. Especially people with lung-disease must go through a transitional stage, which can last several months, during which time some mucus-building substances still have to be taken in to avoid too abrupt, and therefore harmful, a change.

Some of my readers are going to sigh and ask: "What strengthening food can I eat, now that I have to abandon protein-containing meat and leave dried legumes, like peas, lentils, and beans out of my diet?"

I have already stated my opinion on the nutritional value of meat. Our minimal need for proteins can be fully covered by eating sweet fruit. Bananas and nuts, in combination with some figs and dates, build up muscle-mass and offer a fair amount of strength.

Vegetables, chopped up and processed into salads, with oil and plenty of lemons, and all the wonderful fruit, including Mediterranean fruit, are foods worthy of the gods. And when, in springtime, our magnificent fruit, especially apples, become rare, and fresh vegetables are not yet ripe, does Mother Nature not come up with superb oranges from the south? How is it possible that their delicious smell does not make all people want to eat fruit only?

I am not able to go into more detail about diet and

its consequences here. For healthy people this should be enough information to have, and sick people will get specific instructions in regard to their disease and individual condition. I just want to mention that people who do not fast and those who are only slightly sick should at least consider fasting in the mornings. If nothing else, it is quite beneficial to eat nothing but fruit before noon or at least before 10 o'clock. When practiced regularly, small sacrifices like these in one's lifestyle are certain to be rewarded.

3. One last word for those who cannot bring themselves to give up eating the common mucus-containing food (meat, etc.). Even for these people there is a way of eating to health, called "Fletscherism". For this method, proposed by an American named Fletscher, all food is chewed thoroughly until it is liquified. This method though seems to degenerate to a mania lately, and it must be warned against overuse, because otherwise the intestines, used to ballast, will not react anymore and cannot work properly. This method is very useful for sick people in the transition stage to fasting, who cannot bring themselves to abstain from meat, or for certain sicknesses. In America very useful diets with only a little meat and warm water have been developed.

When the person has become healthy (mucus- and germ-free) through fasting and a strict fruit-diet, he no longer has to fast but just has to stick to the fruit-diet. At this state the person will experience eating as a pleasure unknown in life till now. This is the only way for man to find happiness, harmony and the answer to all questions, in particular to the social ones, because only in this manner can man become free of desire and "closer to god" (Socrates).

Can a person constantly live off fruit? Of course!

This doesn't need any proof, otherwise the whole universe would be nonsensical. It would be a "biological error" if every worm could find his food in nature, and only the human species could not. Furthermore there is scientific proof that apples, bananas, and coconuts provide everything nutritional that humans need. A cow lives off grass for its whole life, provides about 10 liters of milk a day, pulls the plough, and finally gets eaten. It produces fat, protein (milk), muscle-mass, strength, and warmth from nothing but metabolizing grass (hay). Understanding such biological basics, would it then follow that this pinnacle animal, the human, is built so awkwardly that his organic life cannot be maintained by food from Mother Nature? Ridiculous.

Nutritional science still erroneously argues that the human body can obtain protein only from fat of animal protein. This is the naïve and unscientific chemical-physiological belief that a substance can only spring from a similar substance. Is it not an absurd thought that a disintegrating protein-molecule of a dead ox's muscle, which is heated in a pan and thus fully "deadened" and then dispersed in the stomach, should—due to a new atomic constellation— revive as a new muscle-molecule in the human body? Weight-gains at so called fattening diets are considered health-gains. One might assume that the unnecessary fattening would cause an increase in muscle-mass, and the sick join in this naiveté. More likely this forced increase in body-weight is a stagnation of ingested fattening food that can no longer be excreted and is a burden on the whole body. Such sick people suffocate gradually in their own, un-excreted residues of their ingested food (fat caused lung disease).

We do not live from what we eat, but from what we

metabolize and assimilate. This assumption is very innovative, but I still have to add much more to it. Our primary life-functions are healthy and work properly as long as we can excrete the excess of food; that is to say we can only temporarily live healthy, not because we metabolize well, but because we excrete the excess food.

Vegetarians, too, have not yet recognized this basic error. The vegetarian protein-supplements have more or less just replaced the inorganic ones that medicine used to provide.

The main downside to fasting is the fact that some people become progressively sicker and weaker, and can even die from unsupervised fasting or fruit-diet. (Obviously, for the vast majority of people, especially the relatively healthy, the opposite occurs.) There is a common opinion that even short fasting weakens the body and that a fruit diet is not sufficient, or that fruit is harder to metabolize than cooked food. Although there is some truth in these observations, the explanation is wrong and misleading. It is not the fasting or the fruit that causes the weakness. Rather, it is the cumulative impact of toxic mucus in the body of sick people, which, through fasting, gets released too quickly. These toxins diffuse into the blood and cause the weakness by essentially re-poisoning the ill person. The cleansing-process has to be slowed down, either by eating a transitional diet or by eating some "decadent delicacies" every now and then.

For an individual who is inherently contaminated by a lifelong protein-diet, by being the child of an alcoholic, or for any other such reason which sadly leads to a cancer or tuberculosis diagnosis, the process of loosening the mucus—even with this most natural of all methods—could be fatal. It is never the fasting and fruit diet itself that harms a person, but the complications associated with the release and elimination of mucus stored in the body.

This is the point where each person must decide for himself whether he wants to go on with obstructing his body and slowly suffocate, or whether he wants to at last take up the challenge of true health by daring to do the unconventional. Even physicians have their boundaries where they declare a person as incurable. Otherwise illness would have no spiritual component. An absolutely regenerated organism eliminates occasionally ingested processed foods as incompatible, which proves once again the necessity of the nature-diet.

III
The True Cause of Aging,
Loss of Attractiveness,
Loss and Graying of Hair

Nature-Based Means for Maintaining Youth and Beauty

After the more general discussions of the preceding chapters concerning mucus as the root cause of illness, I now want to examine the tendency of processed food to decrease the beauty of the human body, causing symptoms of ugliness and premature aging.

If our lungs and skin were provided with pure air only (sun-power), and the gastrointestinal tract had to deal only with fully digestible fruit (sun-food), there would be no reason for the human circulatory system to become defective, lame, or aged, and thus to finally fail. But instead of fruit's living energy cells, people choose to eat "dead chow", biologically designated for carnivores. This is food that has been cooked to death and chemically altered by oxidation (decomposition). It has been robbed of all life energy. The mucus generated by this food concentrates especially in the gastrointestinal tract. Practical experience shows that this mucus is harder to come by with a vegetarian diet, including masses of milk, gruel, rice, potatoes, etc. than with a sensible meat-diet. Over time the cumulative impact of these impurities causes chronic defects, aging, and is the main factor in the etiology of every sickness. Aging is a latent sickness itself, that is to say, a slow but increasing disruption of the body's natural processes.

The chemistry of live food delivers reliable proof that deficiencies of minerals in processed and cooked foods are the sources for deformation and decay in the body.

Can human ugliness, lost beauty and symptoms of age be traced to bad nutrition? If the answer is yes, then a dietetic cure should be the basis for a rejuvenation therapy and beauty restored. As beauty lies in the eye of the beholder and cannot be absolutely defined, I can only stick to the basic norms of aesthetics as I understand them. Although my taste (I am considered an expert in the field of illustration arts) might be in contradiction to that of the general public, at this point I consider it to be quite balanced and based on healthy principles.

I would not consider the deathlike pallor of the lightless and sunless cityfolk as beautiful, especially as it stems mainly from the pale lifeless color of wrong food that has been cooked to death. What a wonderful complexion a person could have if they lived from blood red grapes, cherries and oranges, and if they took regular "air and sun-baths". Not even the modern "Pleinair" (open-air) painters could improve on such a healthful look.

Mucus, with its lack of earth-substances (minerals) causes a lack of color (pallor). Consider the following nutrition tables of Professor Koenig and you will see that the mucus-free food—fruit and vegetables—stand high up in the hierarchy for minerals, especially calcium. The size of a human, that is the development of his bone structure, depends primarily on the amount of calcium in his food. All deformations and abnormalities of bone structure and tooth decay are based on a lack of calcium. It should be noted that calcium is rendered useless in milk and vegetables by the process of cooking them.

The Most Important Foods

Consistency and Units of Nutritional Values

(taken from Koenig, chemistry of human nutritional and comfort foods)

Food	Water	Nitrogen	Fat	Nitrogen-free Substances	Fiber	Minerals
Meat and Meat-products without bones						
Fatty Beef	54.76	18.92	23.65	-	-	1.08
Lean Beef	76.47	20.56	1.74	-	-	1.17
Fatty Veal	72.31	18.88	7.41	0.07	-	1.33
Lean Veal	78.84	19.86	0.82	-	-	0.50
Half-Fatty Mutton	75.99	17.11	5.77	-	-	1.33
Fatty Pork	47.40	14.54	37.34	-	-	0.72
Lean Pork	72.57	20.25	6.81	-	-	1.10
Goose	40.87	14.21	44.26	-	-	0.66
Dove	75.10	22.14	1.00	0.76	-	1.00
Salmon	67.01	19.73	10.74	-	-	1.39
Eel	57.42	12.83	28.37	0.53	-	0.85
Pike	79.84	18.33	0.47	-	-	1.00
Carp	76.97	21.86	1.09	-	-	1.33

Food	Water	Nitrogen	Fat	Nitrogen-free Substances	Fiber	Minerals
Tinned food						
German Sausage (fat)	20.76	39.88	39.88	5.10	-	6.95
Liver Sausage	48.70	26.33	26.33	6.38	-	2.66
Dairy-Products						
Cow-Milk	87.27	3.39	3.68	4.94	-	0.72
Butter	13.45	0.76	83.70	0.50	-	1.59
Fatty Cheese	49.79	18.97	25.87	0.83	-	4.54
Lean Cheese	43.06	35.59	12.45	4.22	-	4.68
Chicken Eggs	73.67	12.55	12.11	0.55	-	1.12
Cereal and Grain						
Rice, plain	13.17	8.13	1.29	75.50	0.88	1.03
Peas	13.80	23.35	1.88	52.65	5.57	2.75
Lentils	12.33	25.94	1.93	52.84	3.92	3.04

Food	Water	Nitrogen	Fat	Nitrogen-free Substances	Fiber	Minerals
Flours, etc.						
Wheat Flour, fine	12.63	10.68	1.13	74.74	0.30	0.52
Wheat Flour, whole	12.58	11.60	1.59	73.39	0.92	1.02
Rye Flour	17.76	0.88	0.05	80.68	0.06	0.57
Macaroni	11.89	10.88	0.62	75.55	0.42	0.64
Bread, etc.						
Fine Wheat Bread	22.66	6.81	0.54	57.80	0.31	0.88
Whole Wheat Bread	37.27	8.44	0.91	50.99	1.12	1.27
Rye Bread	39.70	6.43	1.14	50.44	0.80	1.49
Tubers						
Potatoes	74.93	1.99	0.15	20.86	0.98	1.09
Big Carrot	86.77	1.18	0.29	9.06	1.67	1.03
Celeriac	84.09	1.48	0.39	11.80	1.40	0.84

Food	Water	Nitrogen	Fat	Nitrogen-free Substances	Fiber	Minerals
Leafy Vegetables						
Rutabaga	85.89	2.87	0.21	8.18	1.68	1.17
Onion	86.51	1.60	0.15	10.38	0.71	0.65
Cucumber	95.36	1.09	0.11	2.21	0.78	0.45
Runner Beans	88.75	2.72	0.14	6.60	1.18	0.61
Cauliflower	90.89	2.48	0.34	4.55	0.91	0.83
Kale	80.03	3.99	0.90	11.63	1.88	1.57
Cabbage	90.11	1.83	0.18	5.05	1.65	1.18
Spinach	89.24	3.71	0.50	3.61	0.94	2.00
Lettuce	94.33	1.41	0.31	2.19	0.73	1.03
Sauerkraut	91.41	1.25	0.54	3.85	1.31	1.62
Fruit						
Apples	84.37	0.30	-	12.73	1.98	0.42
Pears	85.83	0.35	-	13.09	0.28	0.29
Plums	81.62	0.78	-	16.76	6.42	1.16
Cherries	80.57	1.29	-	13.63	5.77	0.52

Food	Water	Nitrogen	Fat	Nitrogen-free Substances	Fiber	Minerals
Fruit (cont'd.)						
Grapes	79.12	1.01	-	16.18	3.03	0.48
Strawberries	86.99	0.59	0.53	7.33	1.56	0.72
Walnuts	7.18	16.74	58.47	12.99	2.97	1.65
Sweet Almonds	6.27	21.40	53.16	13.22	3.65	2.30

The terrible lack of minerals contained in processed food (particularly meat) in comparison to fruit, is one of the reasons for generations of toothless people. Even many physicians acknowledge this. Instead of substituting these inadequate foods with fruit, people now augment their insufficient diets with artificial supplements. The human body cannot assimilate such minerals, which are not organic nor derived from plants or fruit.

The latest deformation of the human physique, the modern problem of obesity, has so distorted our aesthetic sense that we no longer even remember the natural baseline of the human form anymore. Obesity comes in many forms. Personally I do not think of the extreme body-builder as the ideal human physique. Weight, form, and bodily volume are too big. Every influence toward obesity is pathological and not at all aesthetic. No free-living animal is so upholstered with fat as these humans. The sole cause is too much food and drink, which leads to sluggishness and constipation of the whole circulatory system. Glucose and mineral salts found in fruit are the truest sources for muscle-mass, which rebuilds a fat-free and mucus-free body after fasting.

Tragically, the tendency and social acceptance of fatness in body and face are increasing dramatically in our society. It is an ugly and pathological development. Equally strange is the fact that this tendency toward obesity is not only considered to be beautiful, but is generally thought to indicate perfect health. Daily experience shows that slender, youthful people are in every sense more robust, and more often reach old age. The scholar Mantegazza long ago noticed that the lean body-type is superior to the fat body-type in strength and endurance, but he did not know why.

The reasons are plain. Just show me one obese person in his 80's or 90's who can eat his way back to health from tuberculosis. How can it be explained that most people in their 100's can be found in the poorest countries, where people are deemed by science to be "malnourished"? If our society's heavily overweight people do not die at the zenith of their lives of a heart attack, stroke or edema, a gradual emaciation starts and the urge for food will diminish. The overly stretched facial skin will become wrinkled, for it has lost its youthful elasticity due to lack of or unhealthy blood supply, not to mention minimal exposure to light and sun. What happens next is that people try to treat the sagging of their skin with topical treatments of lotion and powder. Absurd! Meanwhile, the natural dignity and beauty of the facial traits, the clean and healthy complexion, the clearness and natural size of the eye, the graceful expression and color of the lips—all become old and ugly. Why? Because a lifetime of mucus accretion—the central root-cause of all symptoms, sickness and aging—accumulates in the gastrointestinal tract. The "beautifully fed cheeks" are a manifestation of this slime-constipation that becomes obvious every time we have a runny nose.

I will turn now to the most important and most striking symptom of aging, the loss and graying of hair. I must dedicate a whole part of this chapter to the topic because this phenomenon is usually connected to the biggest anguish that advancing age brings to people. Even science has not solved this puzzle.

We have now become so accustomed to the modern male short-sheared hairstyle and the alarming increase in early baldness that we don't even think about the lack of aesthetics and harmony that this specter of human appearance presents to us. Here we have man, the intellectual and aesthetic "crown of creation", robbed of his own crown, the natural headdress of his hair. "Living Sculls" would be the best term for today's hairless, beardless, pallid heads! Just imagine the most beautiful woman baldheaded! Which man would not back away in fright? Who would want a marble-statue of a modern man, with his geometrically shaped mustache and otherwise beardless face, and his modern clothes, which are distinguished from all clothes of all centuries by their uniform tastelessness? Do we really consider this to be beautiful?

You have to understand the philosophical and historical connections between taste, clothing, architecture and sculpture as a symbolic language of intellect in a particular cultural period, to realize how alarming this deformation of people really is. People, by natural law, should be the most absolutely beautiful and sublime creations of nature. Of course I understand the practical usefulness of the decreased length of beard and shorn head of modern men. The routine lack in beauty and aesthetic appearance of hair and beard has become common enough to naturally bring up an urge for shaving and for millimeter-precise clipping machines. In our time of leveling out and equalization, one would rather cut off those organs of smell and personal disclosure than flaunt ugly, fluffy and uneven hair as living proof of an uncomplimentary theory of ancestry. Considering this, the maltreatment of hair makes sense.

It is easy to draw the conclusion that an unattractive organism is equivalent to a sick organism, i.e., that nature reveals an organism's internal, physiological disturbances and diseases by presenting an outward disharmony in its shapes and colors. Severely sick people and dead organisms are extreme examples of this phenomenon. I want to remind those who doubt this opinion, not to mention those neglectful observers of natural law, of the exception to the rule, and of the fact that society seems to have lost the concept of ideal beauty and health enjoyed by humans who live under absolutely natural circumstances. Just as enjoying beauty has a positive value, the repulsion experienced by the aesthetically trained eye to the ugliness and dissonance of a sick organism's color and shape must stem from some realization of the underlying pathology. When I regard science's incredible eagerness and progress with my professionally artistic eye, I believe that today's world is far too often seen through the microscope instead of the natural eye. For those rigorous and aesthetically oriented observers of nature, the organism's language of color and shape is equivalent to the value of the inner functions, spirit and soul of the organism. The responsibility for the total lack of modern understanding of this must be attributed to the shortcoming of art education at our schools. We face an enormous gap in modern intellectual development that cannot be filled by two or three hours of drawing lessons per week at high school. It is common knowledge among professionals that, with a single word, the most accomplished scholar can be embarrassed in an art gallery in front of the most mediocre art student.

Let us now come back to our topic. We have recognized the modern hairstyle as an unaesthetic disturbance of the generally harmonious perfection of human appearance and we have revealed that badly growing hair is the main reason for this unaesthetic and ugly shape of hair and beard.

Now we have to concern ourselves with the chemical com-
position of hair itself—its physical attributes, and the physiological and biological meaning of hair. In revealing and
coming to understand the true function and importance of
human hair in health and sickness, we can find the causes
for the misunderstood phenomenon of hair loss. This is a
crucial step in pursuing a cure for baldness.

Page 458 of the "Eulenburg" encyclopedia of medical science reads as follows: "The cause for this strange,
universal baldness (Alopekie areata) is yet unknown.
General debilities, anemia, local injuries and the like are
in my opinion not the reason." And on page 459: "The
presence of fungi is repeatedly suggested, but never proved
as an etiological pattern." "The therapy of Alopekie areata
lacks positive empirical basis and is neither able to abbrevi-
ate nor prevent the disease. Worth trying are irritating alcoholic fluids."

From the above, we can see that medicine is power-
less in the face of the disease of baldness. We know that cos-
metics and the hair tonic industry have failed for they have
yet to create even a single new hair. Dr. Anton Reichenow
discusses the consistency of hair in his Encyclopedia of
Natural Science, Volume 4, page 188: "Cornet tissue and
other epidermologic structures (epidermis, hair, nails,
hoofs, claws, talons, feathers, fishbone, tortoise shell, etc.)
consist not only of fat, fatty acids, lecithin, cholesterol, pigments and other inorganic salts of the animal organism,
(such as silica in hair and feathers or copper in colored
feathers), but mainly of albumin (keratin). It is a substance
high in sulfate (silicon 3-8%) contained in human hair that
shows a consistence similar to protein." "Normal hair is a

silical soil-protein"' says chemist Jul. Hensel in "Das Leben" (The Life, page 369).

Reichenow goes on to state in Volume 3 on page 614 regarding the function of hair: "There are two major roles in the importance of hair: a physiological and a biological one. For the physiological function, hair is a passively protecting, warming layer, as hair and the air in between hairs are poor heat conductors. It is known that a cold environment increases the growth of hair."

The biological function is partly covered in the discussion regarding protection above. But more importantly, the biological function includes the active role of hair in relation to the senses of touch and smell. A description of the more active task of hair for insects and hairy animals in general can be found in the works of Fritz Mueller and G. Jaeger. These scientists examine the role of hair as organs of scent, e.g. for male butterflies to spread their "love-charm". G. Jaeger found that all hair has importance as organ of scent in the following way: "While having high absorbencies for chemically musk-like substances that are odoriferous for the individual and its specific species, the substance of hair (especially of mammals) has only low levels of absorbencies for the organism's malodorous evaporations. The absorption is highest at low temperatures and decreases with increasing temperature, relieving some of the scents into the atmosphere. So it is appropriate to speak of a certain odor of hair that creates a atmospheric quality around every being (including humans), which influences every creature who comes close enough to inhale this scented atmosphere. This smell plays an extremely important role in the interrelationships of animals. Its main role is as a "love-charm", the specific scent of the partner's hair in sexual relationships."

This explains too, why some creatures develop special patches of hair either at puberty or every time they rut (called "rutting-hair"). Humans develop pubic hair, beards and hair in their armpits at puberty. This hair plays an important role in courtship, because people know very well, at least instinctually, about its relevance. (An old saying for girls is: A kiss without a beard is like soup without salt.) The development of this positive resonance occurs between creatures of the same species, and in some cases, can cross species lines. A newly purchased dog or horse will develop an immediate liking for its new owner if fed some of its owner's hairs. This technique is commonly employed by practitioners of natural living who, through knowledge, not superstition, induce the development of closeness due to the "love-scent' via scenting of the atmosphere, and also by licking, kissing or ingestion of hair. The scent is of course more intense with a big amount of highly developed hair and an increased body-temperature.

G. Jaeger also discusses a corollary practice employed by native peoples, as well as naturopaths and physicians in former centuries (e.g. Paracelsus): The hair-scent is not only a general aphrodisiac, like musk, but acts also as an animal's personal healing agent. It is a tool for self-healing employed by the creature that generates it, and is a powerful elixir, as or more effective than specific remedies of herbal medical science, when used by other creatures. G. Jaeger suggests that the secret of success of modern magnetizers, also called "healing-magnetism" or "life-magnetism", is nothing more or less than the individual scent, supplied in skin tallow, epidermis tissue, and hair grease. G. Jaeger had introduced this scent into his healing-techniques, called "Anthropie".

Dr. Joh. Ranke mentions the consistency and build-up of hair in his book "Der Mensch" (The Human). On page 160 he writes: "Sulfur in hair rubs off so easily that even touch with lead blackens the hair. The main source of hair color are the outer layers of hair." And on page 163: "The lifespan of head hair is, according to Pinos, two to four years. Surprisingly baldness is more likely for men than for women.1 " On page 165: "According to studies
by Berthold, hair grows faster in daytime than nighttime, and also grows faster during the warm season. Shaving accelerates the growth of hair—beards grow twice as fast if shaved every 12 hours instead of every 36 hours." And finally on page 171: "European peoples, due to cultural dis-advantages, have the highest number of bald or gray-haired people, and the graying of hair starts earliest on average.

A. v. Humboldt's observation is relevant here. He said: "Travelers who judge Indian physiognomy could be led to think that this culture has scarcely any old people. It is really hard to estimate the native's age without reading their town's birth register, which, by the way, is made more difficult because they are devoured by termites every 20 to 30 years. They themselves, the poor Indian country-people in New-Spain, usually do not know how old they are. Their hair does not turn gray, and it is indefinitely rare to find an Indian or Negro with white hair. Furthermore their skin does not wrinkle easily, and often natives in Mexico, espe-cially the women, live up to their 100's. Mexican and Peruvian Indians usually live into high age keeping their bodily strength up to death." Humboldt goes on to mention a native Indian who lived to be 143 years old and up to his 130th year he walked three to four hours daily.

I will now examine some details about the build-up of head hair, which is as microscopically structured as any other fiber in the human body.

Every day a hair grows 0.2 – 0.3 mm. Fallen out hair grows back quickly, as long as the papillae are alive. The length of all hair that has ever been cut off in a man's life taken together would be 11 to 14 meters. This fact proves how much this unostensive organ means to nature. One should also think about the amounts of good and important substances that the body has to activate in order to replace the cut off pieces. I long ago meditated on this problem at the age of 16. My father was shaved two hours prior to his death, and until the day of his funeral, three days later, his beard grew back as strong as usual. The contraction of skin and facial muscles at rigor mortis is not sufficient as an explanation for this strange phenomenon. Similar observations have been made at exhumations of dead people. As I do not have any reliable evidence for these observations I would be very grateful for information on this matter.

For discouraged and hopeless bald-heads I want to mention some interesting and scientifically based facts: Eulenburg, Medical Real-encyclopedia, 1896, Volume 3, page 363: "According to Albert, a woman suffering from nervous puerperal fever, lost her blond hair and black hair grew back. In another case a brunette woman lost her hair during an illness and flaming red hair grew back. The gray hair of a 66-year old woman is said to have turned black shortly prior to her death."

Geigel stated that a woman developed black hair instead of her blond hair, which had fallen out when she suffered from black typhus."

I am in perfect agreement with Prof. Dr. Jaeger. I think of hair, especially human head hair, as the scent-organs of the human body, dissipating bodily evaporations. Everybody knows that we perspire first on our heads and in the armpits, and that the sweat of sick people is connected with an unpleasant smell. This is also the reason why Prof. Dr. Jaeger refers to sickness as "malodorousness". All of this seems correct to me, especially as I postulate the following general terms of sickness, referring to observations and experiments that I have conducted over many years.

Sickness is a process of the body's deterioration and decomposition, or of the excretion of mucus caused by the ingestion of excessive and unnatural foods and their cumulative buildup in the digestive organs over time.

Basically sickness is a chemical decay or disintegration of cellular protein. This process is accompanied by stench, while nature usually associates the creation of new life with fragrance (florescence of plants). The perfectly healthy human, especially his hair, should diffuse fragrance. Poets have rightly compared humans with flowers and talk about the wonderful scent of women's hair. I perceive people's hair as an important organ which protects and regulates the body-temperature, and which evaporates the scent of healthy and sick people. It allows appreciators to make judgements about a person's qualities and determine a person's inner health or sickness. While physicians are not able to diagnose disorders of digestion using microscopes and testing tubes, some "charlatans" are able to determine the smelly process of internal decay using the simple hair-diagnosis. Today, even adolescents, who seem to be perfectly healthy and strong, suffer from horrible halitosis and are surprised to have their hair begin to gray and to lose it.

At this point I must say a few more words about the graying of hair. As already mentioned, the content of air increases in graying hair, and I assume that this "air" consists at least partly of stinking gases. I suggest for clever chemists to search for a sulphurous acid here, which would also explain the decrease of pigments in the hair, as it is common knowledge that sulfur dioxide bleaches.

I am perfectly sure, especially because of my numerous interesting experiments with my own body, that the main cause for the loss of hair can only be an internal one. It is not surprising that the whole hair including hair roots becomes pale, dies and falls out if we consider that the hairs, the "scent-pipes" (the "exhaust-chimneys") constantly have to discharge gases that are stinky, acrid and very likely full of sulfur dioxide, instead of natural, scented fragrances. With this explanation I claim to have found the cause of baldness, and to have shown an unmistakable way to cure it. The photographs printed in the appendix, underpin my assumptions. I have to add that my hair was severely graying and falling out during the time of the chronic inflammation of my kidneys, which was accompanied by severe anxiety (picture 3). After I started my dietary healing process and got cured from my severe illness, the gray in my hair, too, decreased and my hair grew back gorgeously (picture 8).

Given the main causes for hair loss are disorders of digestion and metabolism, it follows that only through those areas can there be alleviation of symptoms. I believe that these findings can give hope, even to absolutely bald people, after the failures of hair tonic. As the cause is not an external one it cannot be eliminated from the outside. It can even be unhealthy to use too many hair products, as many contain pungent, inorganic substances (like some hair-dyes) and can therefore be harmful. Only herbal hair tonics, like nettle tinctures, can be of any positive use to the hair. This is true, not because of the nettle components per sé, but because of the odoriferous and aerial herbs and the fatty substances included, which resemble in scent the natural, healthy, youthful growth of hair. I am more than willing to advise those who already lose hair or suffer from baldness. There is no general panacea, and those who understand my argument will understand that individual advice is needed. With the influence of my diet on metabolism and blood development I can guarantee the right nourishment of the skull and the solution to even the worst loss of hair if my advice is followed correctly.

I suggest to every intelligent researcher to read "Entdeckung der Seele" (Discovery of the Soul) by Prof. Dr. Jaeger. This book offers a natural science introduction into the world of scents which, in my opinion, illuminates secrets, like diet and the life of soul and sex. Beautiful hair is not only a major factor of fancy and attraction, but is mainly a manifestation of unfolding, blooming life, just like the blooming of flowers. Today's dismaying number of bald people has to be seen as a symptom of the decreasing strength of the individual and the decline of a people. Full and lustrous hair is not only the sign of youthful life and strength, but it also strengthens the life's energy. I deliver living proof that even for people close to death a rebirth is possible.

All symptoms of aging are latent sicknesses, accumulations of mucus and circulation problems caused by mucus. Everyone who goes through a healing cure after any sickness and eats a mucus-free diet, or fasts to rid his body of dead cells, gets a more youthful appearance and deprives every sickness of its basis. As self-evident as this is, few want to believe in this possibility. The assumptions postulated in lexicons are that the only disease-free way for people to die would be of disorders in their metabolism (mucus-based constipation). Unfortunately this is rather the exception to the rule and illness is the more common case. If people would eat only fruit from young age on they would not age or become sick. I have known people who, over time, became so much more youthful and beautiful due to the mucus-free diet that I did not recognize them at first.

For thousands of years people have been dreaming of the fountain of youth, have written poems about it, painted pictures of it and searched for it in the stars and in their imagination.

How much money do we spend uselessly on remedies for impotence and infertility? And how easy would it be to cure those illnesses, just by the right, pleasurable food from the sun-kitchen.

We can only guess how much beauty and skills the "godlike" human being in paradise possessed; what a wonderfully strong and clear voice he had. The beautifying and strengthening of the voice, the regaining of the lost voice, is a baffling symptom of my cure, which speaks for itself and the great impact that my system has on the whole organism of the sick person. I want to point out the wonderful effect that my cure had in the case of the Bavarian singer Heinrich Knote in Munich. He himself talks about this in his letter of thanks that is printed in the appendix: "… my voice, growing in strength and vividness …" and the "Muenchner Zeitung writes in its review of Knote's "Tannhaeuser" on March 18, 1911: "The radical vegetarianism (the absolutely mucus-free diet) seems to do the singer good. His beautiful, flexible, technically exemplary educated voice sounded clear and healthy, fresh and youthfully strong, often powerfully overflowing. His approach to the tones was light, safe and apparently effortless, a legato, a guiding of air, such as otherwise only found in Caruso. And this master-tenor is thereby a lot more than a tenor … ."

I want to finish this chapter with a citation from
Goethe's Faust I:

Mephistopheles:
>My friend, now you are talking wisely.
>For your rejuvenation there is a natural means;
>Only it is written in a different book
>And is a strange chapter.

Faust: I want to know it.

Mephistopheles: Well, then! A means, available without
>Any physician or magic:
>Go on out into the field,
>Start hacking and digging,
>Maintain yourself and your senses
>In a very limited circle
>Eat only unmilled food,
>Live with the beasts as a beast, and do not
>slaughter them
>Work the land yourself from which you harvest;
>This is the best means
>To rejuvenate yourself another eighty years!

Faust: I am not used to this, and I cannot convince myself,
>To take the spade into my hand.
>This narrow life does not fit me.

Mephistopheles: Well, then we have to resort to witchcraft!

Page 91. This photo is from the cover of a 1914 edition of Kranke Menschen from which this book was translated. Ehret first published Kranke Menschen in 1910. The 1914 edition was the third and last edition of Kranke Menschen in German. In the 1914 edition there were probably some small changes in the text from the first edition. This cover is believed to be the same cover as the first edition cover.

Page 92. This photo is from the beginning of the 1914 edition of "Kranke Menschen". It shows the sanitarium that was practicing and teaching Ehret's Mucusless Diet Healing System. The building still exists in Lugano - Massagno, Switzerland. Today it looks the same as in this photo. It is now a well kept six-family apartment building. There is no trace of a group of people following Ehret's teachings in Canyonville, Oregon.

Page 93. This page came after and faced the page that the sanitarium was on. It is the cover page for the book.

Page 94. This is a copy of Ehret's Preface to "Kranke Menschen".

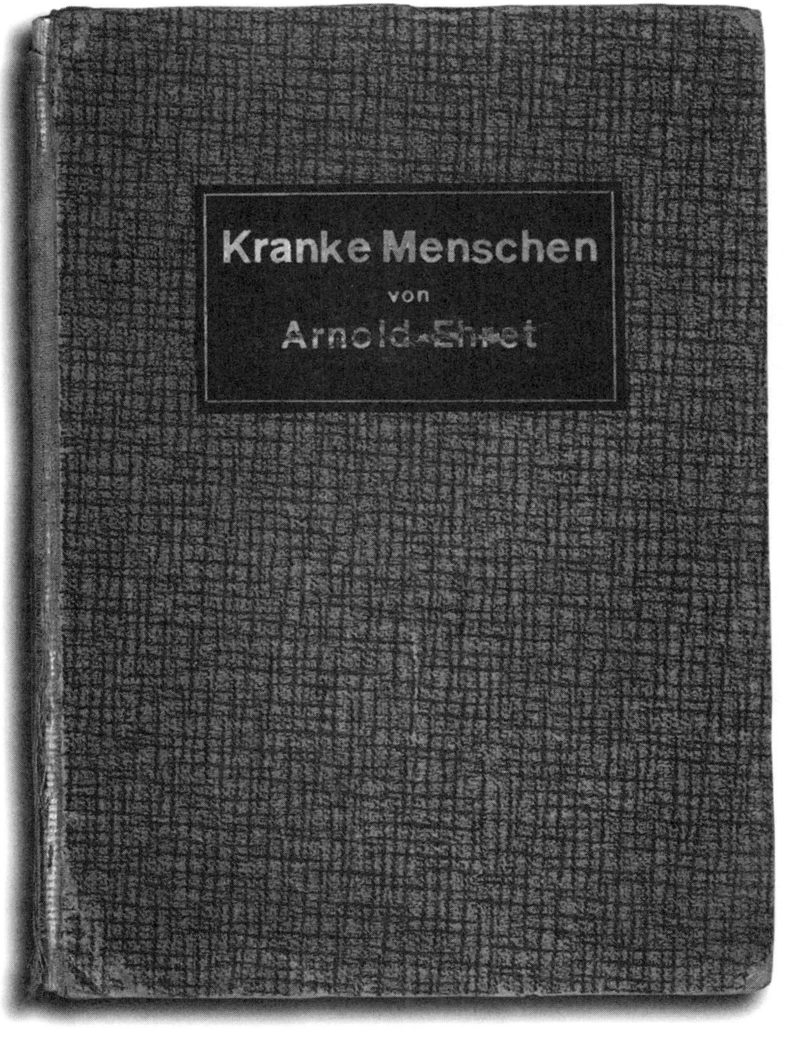

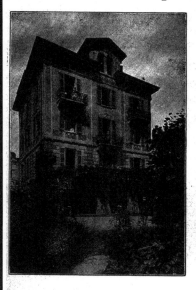

KRANKE MENSCHEN

Der gemeinsame Grundfaktor im Wesen aller Krankheiten, des Alterns und des Todes

von

ARNOLD EHRET.

9. bis 12. Tausend.

Es hat einmal ein Tor gesagt,
Der Mensch sei zum Leiden geboren,
Seitdem ist dies — Gott sei's geklagt,
Der Spruch aller leidenden Toren.
Mirza Schaffy.

1914.

EHRET-VERLAG MÜNCHEN
(in Kommission bei Carl Kuhn Verlag, München).

Vorwort

Ein Teil der vorliegenden Arbeit ist im Jahre 1910 in der „Gesundheit", Zürich, und in Nr. 17/18 der „Lebenskunst", Verlag K. Lentze, Leipzig, als Aufsatz erschienen und erregte solches Aufsehen und eine derartige Nachfrage, daß ich mich veranlaßt sehe, sie in wesentlich erweiterter Form und mit wichtigen Ergänzungen versehen zu veröffentlichen.

Möge diese Schrift den Menschen, die Wahrheit suchen, von wem sie auch komme, und besonders den Kranken dienen und eine Anregung sein für solche, denen die entschwindende Jugend und die Symptome des Alterns Sorge machen.

Schon nach Jahresfrist ist das 5. Tausend von „Kranke Menschen" vergriffen, ein Beweis, welchen Anklang das Buch gefunden hat. Möge mit der 2. Auflage die Wahrheit, die es vertritt, sich weitere Bahnen öffnen. Einige kleinere Ergänzungen wurden vorgenommen, sonst blieb der Inhalt des Buches unverändert.

Locarno, Herbst 1912.

Arnold Ehret.

Page 96. This is a photo taken in Canyonville, Oregon circa 1919. It is the camp where Ehret was staying in Canyonville. Ehret is on the right in front of the tent.

Page 97. This photo shows Ehret sitting at the campsite with friends. From left to right – unknown person probably Watzig, Ehret and John Edgar Marx. Marx was Hans Schmidt until World War I when he changed his name. He apparently did it because of malice against Germans because of the war. He was living in the United States during the war.

Page 98. This is an enlargement of Ehret from the Canyonville, Oregon campsite photo.

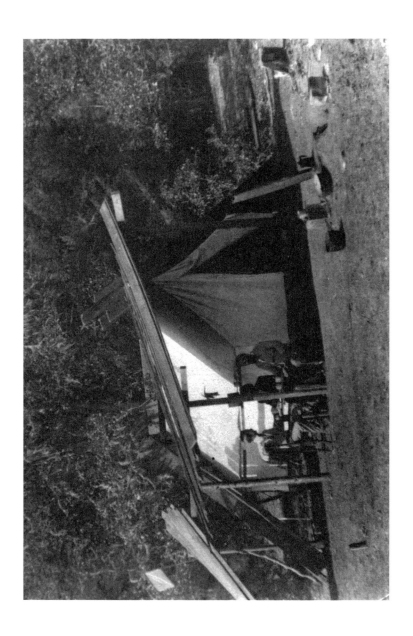

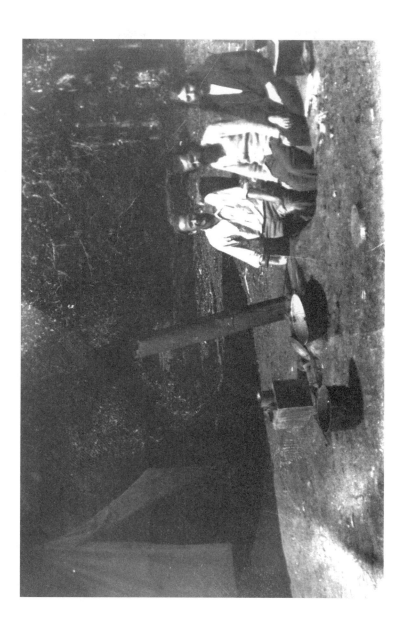

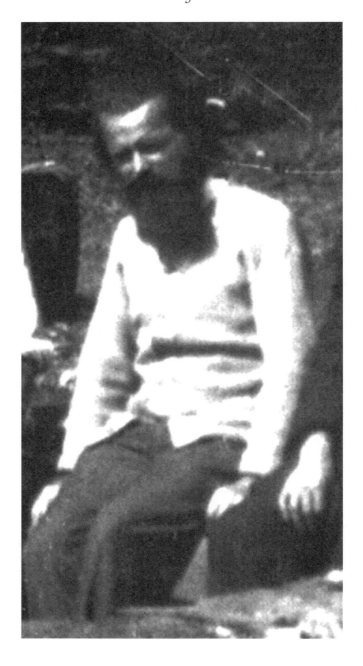

Page 100. This is a photo of the graduation banquet of the Mucusless Diet Healing System Course held on July 6, 1922. It was called the Practitioners Graduating Class. This picture seems to contain the first reference to the word Ehretists for people who follow Ehret's teachings. Fred Hirsch is the only person other than Ehret who is identifiable in the picture. Hirsch is sitting to the right of Ehret. Hirsch was his patient, his business associate and a graduate of the Mucusless Diet Healing System Course, Class of 1921. Hirsch died in 1979.

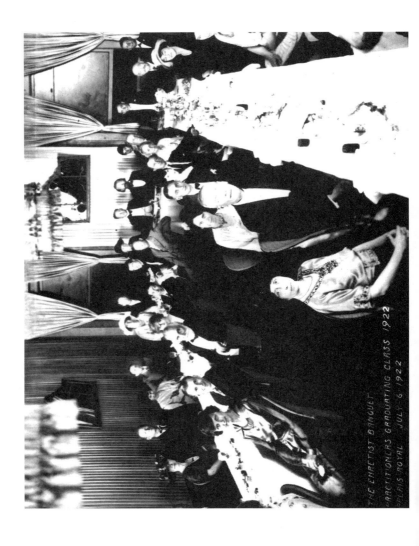

THE EMPETIST BANQUET
PRACTITIONERS GRADUATING CLASS 1922
...ELAIS ROYAL   JULY 6 1922

The next two pages have a group of pictures from what Ehret called his "eight photographs". Two of them, Photograph 3 and 8, are mentioned in this book. However, he did not put any of them in the 1914 edition of "Kranke Menschen". The next eight photographs are from the original studio photographs.

Page 102 contains photographs 1 through 4.

Page 103 contains photographs 5 through 8

Page 104. This photograph was taken during his short military career. It was taken in München (Munich), Germany, circa 1882.

Page 105. This photograph, circa 1894, was taken when he was 28 years old. The way he dressed appears that he came from at least a middle class family.

Page 106 and 107. The photograph and the tissue that covered the photograph, on the following page, have a date of 1895. He was 29 years old. He would resume teaching at the University two years later.

Page 108. This photograph is circa 1908 when he was starting to grow a full beard.

Page 109. This photograph was taken in mid 1909. He has changed his appearance by letting his beard grow out.

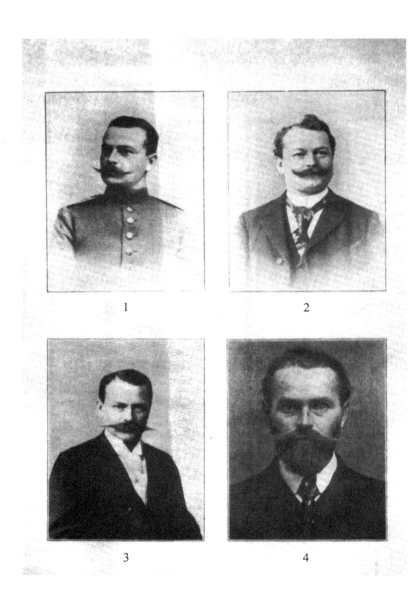

1

2

3

4

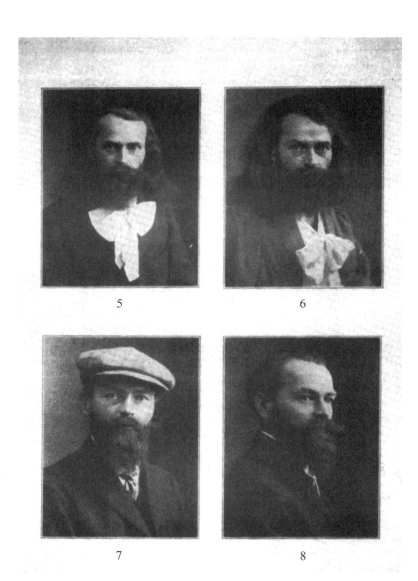

5

6

7

8

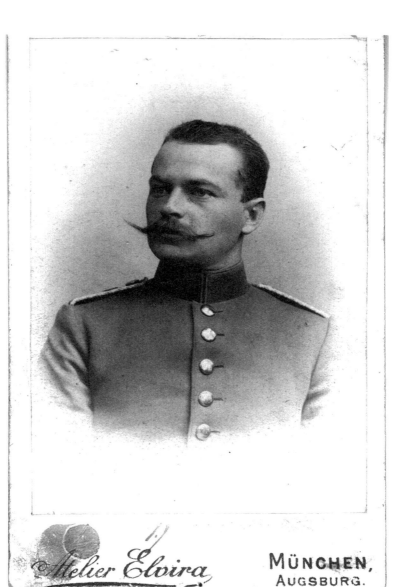

Atelier Elvira   MÜNCHEN,
                                  AUGSBURG.

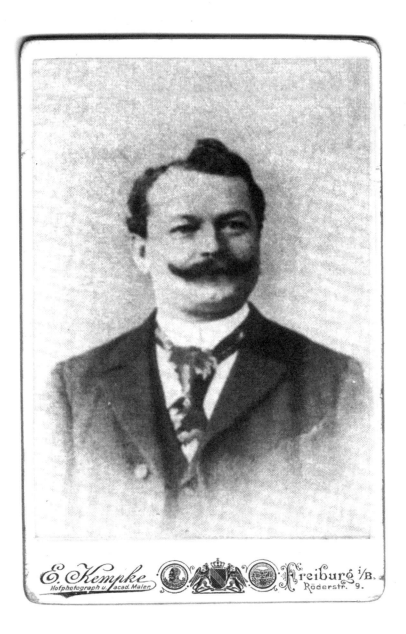

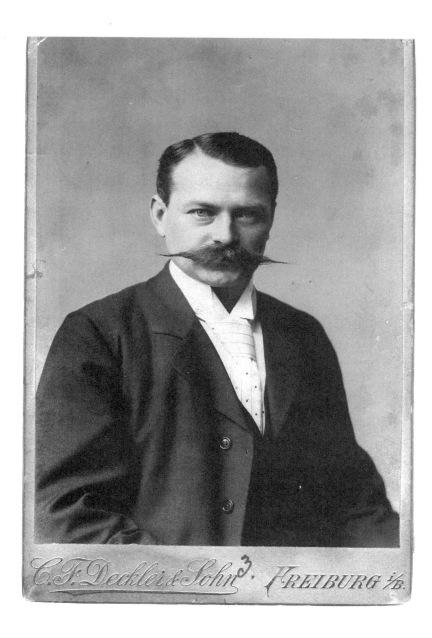

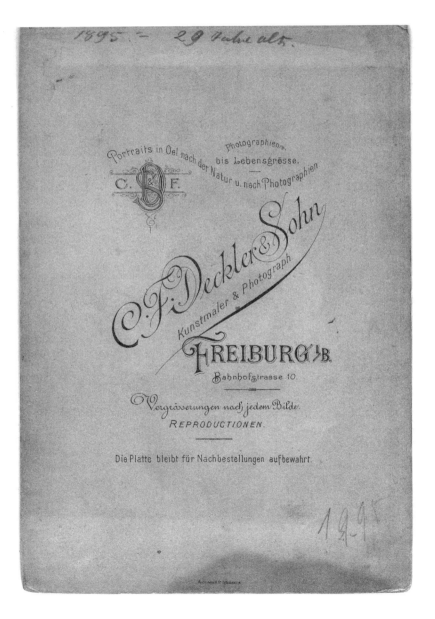

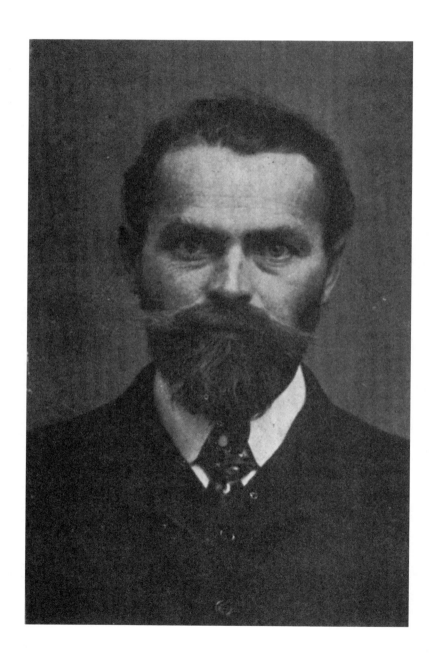

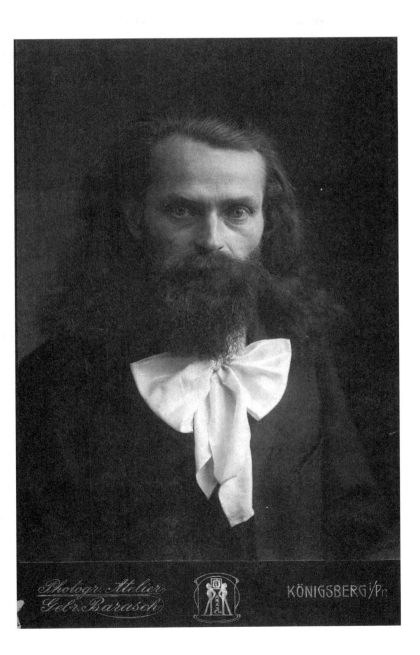

Page 111. This photograph was taken in 1909 probably after the photograph on the previous page. These two photographs show how his features changed in a short period of time as he was testing his Mucusless Diet on himself.

Page 112. This photograph, circa 1913, was taken when he was involved with a nudist health movement in Ascona, Switzerland at Villa Monte Verita.

Page 113. This photograph, circa 1915, was the last photograph we know of, taken before he came to the United States in 1917.

Page 114 and 115. These body building photographs were probably taken during his eleven months of military service. They were taken in München (Munich), Germany circa 1882. He appears to be in good physical condition even though he was released from service for medical reasons.

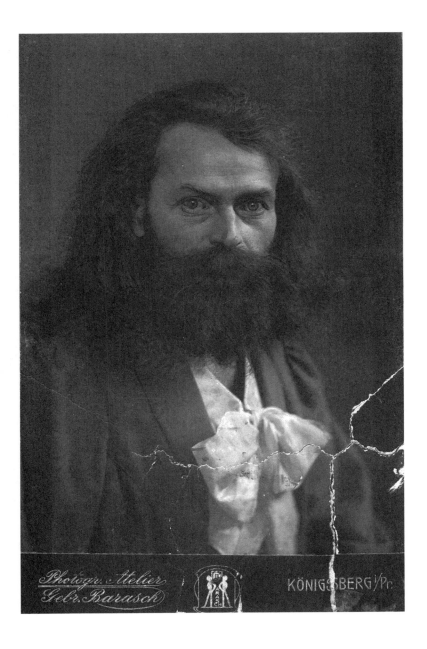

Photogr. Atelier
Gebr. Barasch

KÖNIGSBERG i/Pr.

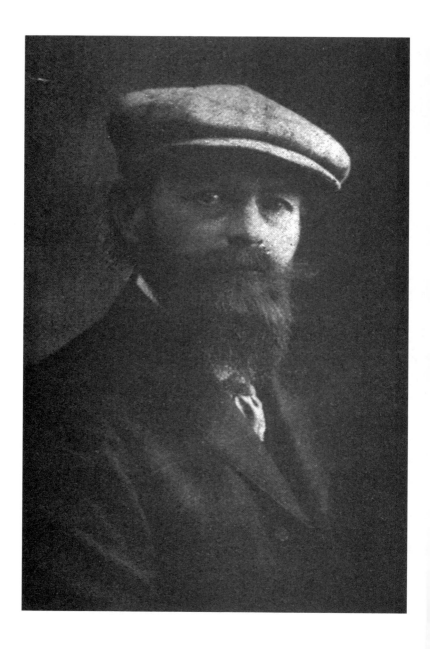

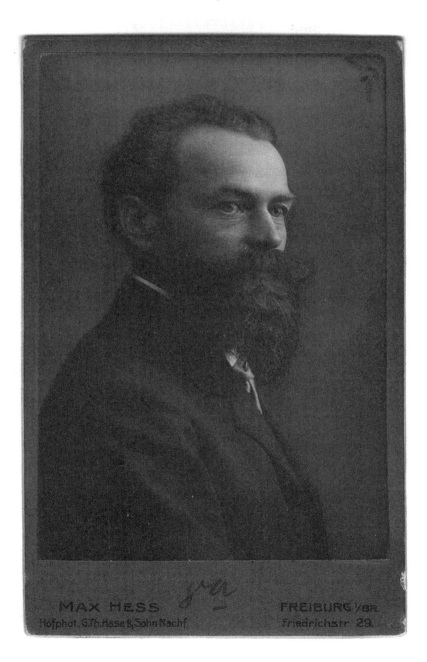

MAX HESS   FREIBURG i/br.
Hofphot. G.Th. Hase & Sohn Nachf.   Friedrichstr. 29.

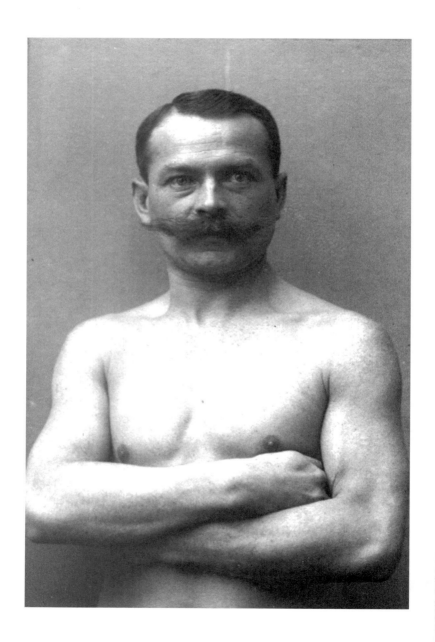

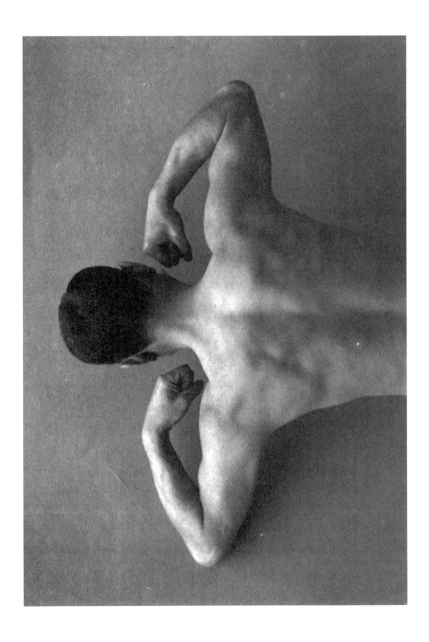

Page 117. Ehret held his lectures and Mucusless Diet Healing System Course classes in Los Angeles, California. This is one of the diplomas which he called certificates. Ehret produced them himself, in watercolors, for his graduating classes. Ehret was an artist, taught art and was a Professor of Art at a university is Munich, Germany. This certificate was given to Fred Hirsch, a graduate of the Class of 1921. The torch shown on the diploma is a symbol of the "Torch of Learning". He later changed it to look like the torch below.

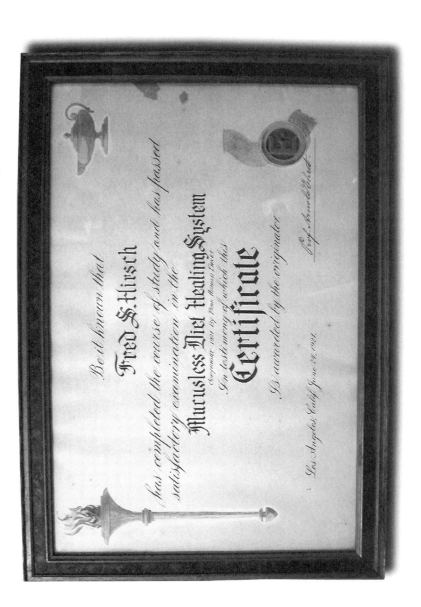

Be it known that

Fred S. Hirsch

has completed the course of study and has passed
satisfactory examination in the

Mucusless Diet Healing System

Copyright 1922 by Prof. Arnold Ehret

In testimony of which this

Certificate

Is awarded by the originator

Prof. Arnold Ehret

Los Angeles, Calif. June 24, 1921.

Page 119. This is a copy of Ehret's birth certificate. He was born in St. Georgen (Saint George) a suburb of Freiburg in the southern part of Germany on July 29, 1866.

Page 120. This is a copy of a postcard from Freiburg, Germany at the turn of the nineteenth century.

Page 121. This is a copy of the advertisement Ehret ran in the Los Angeles Times on October 8, 1922. It would become the last "FREE LECTURE!" Ehret would give. He fell and sustained a skull fracture when leaving the hotel when the lecture was over. He died almost immediately after falling.

Page 122. This copy of Ehret's death certificate states the date of his death as October 10th. He actually died very late in the evening, after the lecture, on October 9th.

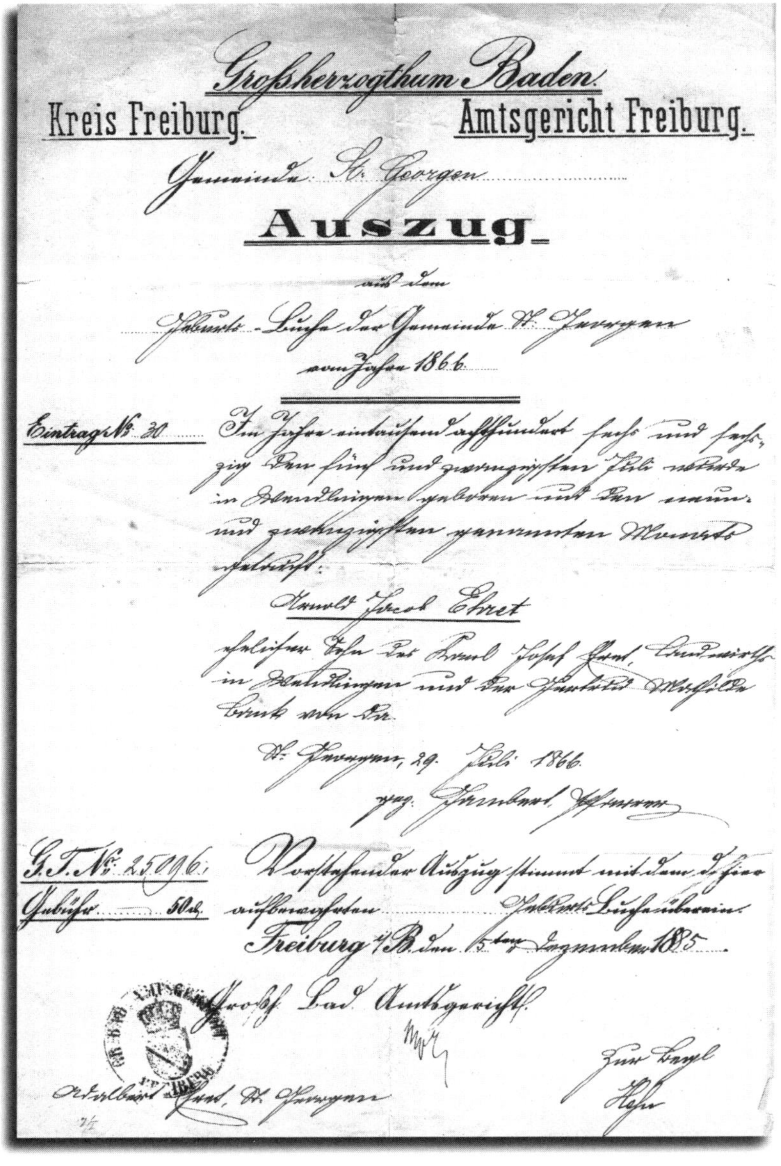

Großherzogthum Baden.

Kreis Freiburg. Amtsgericht Freiburg.

Gemeinde St. Georgen

Auszug.

aus dem

Geburts-Buche der Gemeinde St. Georgen

vom Jahre 1866.

Eintrag No 30 Im Jahre eintausend achthundert sechs und sechzig den fünf und zwanzigsten Juli wurde in Wendlingen geboren und den neun und zwanzigsten genannten Monats getauft:

Arnold Jacob Ehret

ehelicher Sohn des Karl Josef Ehret, Landwirths in Wendlingen und der ...

St. Georgen, 29. Juli 1866.

G.T. No 25096. Vorstehender Auszug stimmt mit dem dahier

Gebühr 50 d. aufbewahrten Geburts Buche überein.

Freiburg i/B. den 5ten Dezember 1885

Großh. bad. Amtsgericht.

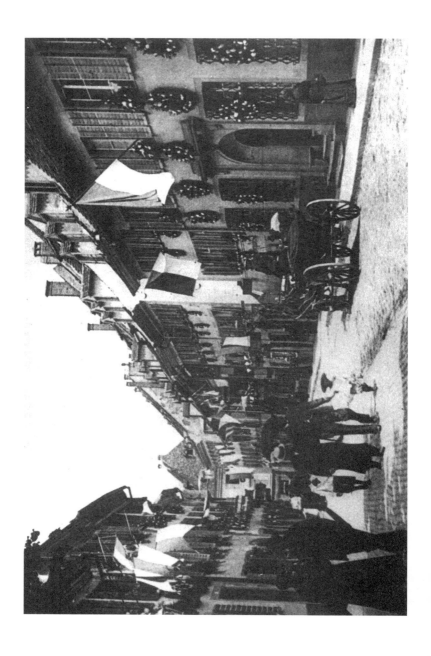

FREE LECTURE!

"THE DIAGNOSIS OF YOUR DISEASE AND HOW TO HELP YOURSELF"

A Momentous Message by

Prof. ARNOLD EHRET

Originator of the MUCUSLESS DIET HEALING SYSTEM

ANGELUS HOTEL — ASSEMBLY HALL

Second Floor, 4th and Spring Sts., MONDAY, OCT. 9, at 8 p.m.
The public is cordially invited.

The lecture will be preceded by a talk and demonstration by MRS. W. S. WILKE WITH HER CHILDREN.

Dr. Henry Gross, Dr. Harry M. Gifford and other practitioners will also speak.
Mail Address. 404 S. Palm Ave., Alhambra, Cal.

STATE OF CALIFORNIA
CERTIFICATION OF VITAL RECORD

COUNTY OF LOS ANGELES • REGISTRAR-RECORDER/COUNTY CLERK

California State Board of Health
BUREAU OF VITAL STATISTICS
STANDARD CERTIFICATE OF DEATH

State Index No. ____
Local Registered No. **7904**

PLACE OF DEATH, DIST. No. ____
County of ____
City or Town of ____
or Rural Registration District ____
(No. ____ Receiving Hospt. ____ St.; ____ Ward)

FULL NAME ARNOLD EHRET

PERSONAL AND STATISTICAL PARTICULARS

SEX: Male
COLOR OR RACE: Cauc.
SINGLE, MARRIED, WIDOWED, OR DIVORCED: Single

DATE OF BIRTH: July — 1866
AGE: 56 years

OCCUPATION: Teacher of Dietetics

BIRTHPLACE: Germany
NAME OF FATHER: Unknown
BIRTHPLACE OF FATHER: Germany
MAIDEN NAME OF MOTHER: Unknown
BIRTHPLACE OF MOTHER: Germany

LENGTH OF RESIDENCE
In California: 5 years

THE ABOVE IS TRUE TO THE BEST OF MY KNOWLEDGE
Informant: Fred Hirsch
Address: 846 E. 6th St.
Filed Oct. 11 1922

CORONER'S CERTIFICATE OF DEATH

DATE OF DEATH: Oct. 10 1922

THE CAUSE OF DEATH was as follows:
Fracture of skull, accidental.
Fell and struck head on curbing.

(Signed) Approved: Frank A. Nance
By Wm. M. Durkin, Jr. Coroner
October 11 1922

PLACE OF BURIAL OR REMOVAL: Forest Lawn Crematory
DATE OF BURIAL: 10-11-22
UNDERTAKER: Booth & Boylson Co.
ADDRESS: 1147 S. Flower St.
EMBALMER'S LICENSE No. 1485

Conny B. McCormack
Registrar-Recorder/County Clerk

ANY ALTERATION OR ERASURE VOIDS THIS CERTIFICATE

Page 124. This is a map of Forest Lawn Memorial Park in Glendale, California where Ehret's ashes are kept in a bronze urn. The mausoleum the urn is in is not accessible to the general public because many famous movie stars remains are there. This is not the famous Forest Lawn Memorial Park – Hollywood. The Hollywood Park did not exist in 1922.

Page 125. This is a photo of the bronze acorn urn in Forest Lawn Memorial Park - Glendale that contains Ehret's ashes. The urn is on view in a glass-fronted cubicle.

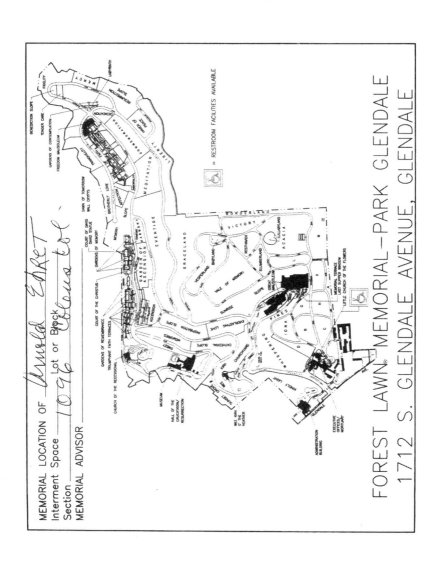

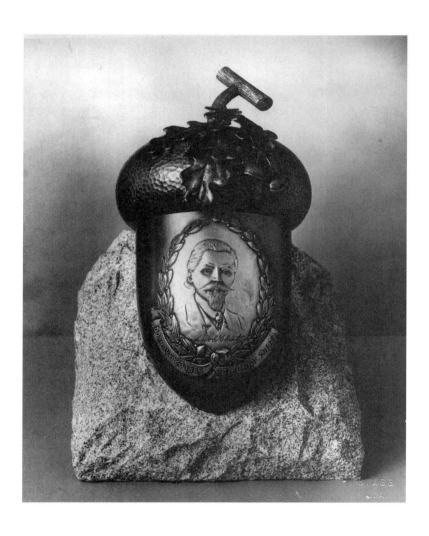

127. Ehret's "Intestinal Broom", an herbal laxative, developed and blended by him personally to assist with fasting and colon cleansing and to help with his Mucusless Diet Healing System's Transition Diet. He called his "Intestinal Broom" Innerclean®. The following photo of an Innerclean delivery truck indicates another way used to support Ehret's teachings. He is said to have charged $100.00 for his Mucusless Diet Healing System course. This was a very large amount of money at that time.

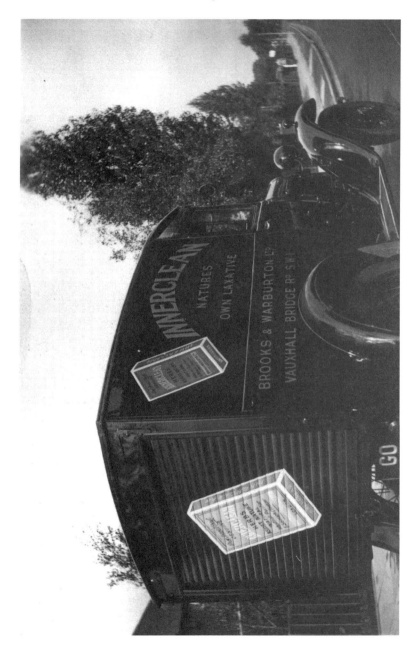

IV
Death

In the preceding chapters mucus has been identified and established as the main cause of illness and aging. I have also proved the possibility of replacing dead cells. In consideration of these facts it cannot be denied that the complete cessation of the human motor can be postponed for a very long time, if the body has been raised and maintained with living sunfood from childhood on. In any case, the sunfood-nourished body has a tremendous advantage over the junkfood-body because its basic elements are much more durable. An optimal lifestyle will reduce the metabolism significantly. The stress on the inner organs, especially the heart and the stomach, will be much less. A mucus-less organism achieves athletic peak performances with a much lower pulse frequency than a glutton. If we include the daily reduction in wasted energy—the continuous decrease in necessary power output—into a longevity equation, we can calculate and prove mathematically an extension of life. But now the question arises whether the removal of all mucus and therefore the removal of cell disease can free us from the ultimate illness, the final mystery of death.

When a person suffers from life-threatening injuries or illness, it is the heart and the brain whose malfunctioning finally leads to death. One can even say that most diseases involve, in their last stages, heart complications. There is still much research to be done in this area, but we can ascertain at this point that a clogging of the coronary blood vessels leading to a weakening of the heart muscle, and the distinction of the fine nerves in the heart due to a constant retoxification of the blood, is the final cause of death in all chronic illnesses. The same is true for the clogging of the tiny capillaries in the brain and the breaking of these blood-vessels in the case of stroke or a major artery blockage, which brings all other life-functions to an abrupt end. Of course there may be secondary causes involved, e.g. insufficient oxygen due to a malfunctioning lung, etc. Medical science also claims the proliferation of white blood cells as a cause of death. This process is called leukemia, which actually translates literally as 'white blood'. I interpret this condition as a severe imbalance where there is more mucus than blood. There is a host of other causes of death, which have been identified: autointoxication, metabolic toxins, external poisons, bacteria and their waste, retoxification, poisons from alcohol and meat as temperance advocates and vegetarians claim. But these abstinent people still die from many diseases, and in doing so they display the same rarely less painless symptoms as the alcoholic and the meat-eater.

If no clear diagnosis can be attributed as the cause of death, the death certificate usually lists "Cachexia" which sounds very scientific, but actually means 'bad condition, decay, malnutrition'. My question is: Which toxin causes death? Medical science sees bacteria as the cause of most diseases. It obviously shares my view that a common foundation factor is involved in aging and death, and undoubtedly a large portion of the myriad of symptoms and conditions can be attributed to bacteria. My empirical proof for mucus being the etiological main and causative factor differs from germ theory only in so far as I view the mucus as the precondition, the receptive terrain, the primary element.

The predominance of the white blood cells, which means a predominance of the dead white mucus, over the red glucose and iron substance in the body becomes a fatal imbalance. Red and sweet are the sensory symbols for life and love; white, colorless, pale and bitter are the indicators of disease and the predominance of mucus, signs of the slow death of the individual. It is pure blasphemy to natural law, yet typical for our culture to interpret the "noble paleness", this complexion of the average city person, as beautiful and healthy. Even art has defiled its aesthetics with this misconception.

The final battle with death is actually only a last attempt of the organism to expel mucus; a final fight of living cells to defeat the dead cells and their toxins. If the white, dead cells gain the upper hand, if the mucus in the blood prevails, then there is not only physiological clogging of the heart arteries, but a chemical transformation, a complete and sudden toxification, a total sepsis and the organism stands still. After death we assign the ultimate cause back to God or fate and say: "It was God's will." or "We capitulate before the mysterious power of death."

"Ignorance is the only tragedy of life. There is no other.", says Peter Altenberg in his book "Prodromos". The ultimate cause of all diseases, aging and unnatural death is a form of spiritual ignorance, a sin we commit unknowingly and for which we pay the ultimate penalty while pleading innocent. But in nature as in civil law ignorance does not absolve us from responsibility.

The purpose of my work is to make a contribution to the war against ignorance, this fatal pitfall for so many suffering human beings, and to disseminate knowledge, which will be a true blessing for every individual and all people, for everybody and all souls.

V
Epilogue

What is simple and obvious by nature has assumed the proportions of the incredible to modern man. He has lost the trust in his own senses and faith and is now lost in the labyrinth of scientific theories. Art is in the process of returning to simplicity and therefore may recover true beauty. Let us hope that we can also return to genuine and truthful understanding. Truth is and must be simple, so it can be understood directly without elaborate schemes of proof. Even if we lack faith, truth always comes in simple, ordinary solutions, as Goethe earlier pointed out.

Some of my readers may find it useful to hear some evaluations of experts and read some medical documentation about my experiential research. Before I present these I would like to talk to my readers about a series of photographs of me. Their sequential progression demonstrates quite clearly the physiognomic transformations I went through since my youth. These pictures document how I descended into serious illnesses and regained total health. Nature wants to regenerate us through the process of illness. Nature wants us to go through a genuine rebirth, to guide us to a physical resurrection in the deepest sense of the word. If you want to rejuvenate yourself, before becoming ill, then you must engage voluntarily in fasting and eating living foods (especially fruit). It is only after all poisons—everything bad, foul and dead—has been expelled, that nature begins to build a new, rejuvenated human being upon the remaining foundation of basically intact cells. It makes sense of course that the body looks old and terrible during this process of detoxification and purification.

But what will we do with the cattle, pigs and chickens? What will happen to the butchers and brewers? Even the bakers will be ruined! This purification and rejuvenation will cause a stock market crash! Many of my readers ask such frightening questions. But please, relax. Such worries are completely unfounded. Even if our whole society went through a process of detoxification, the transition would happen so slowly that no business would have to close. Such a transformation would take thousands of years and, in actuality, I do not believe in the realistic possibility of complete collective change. There will be no paradise regained on planet earth. All political entities in this world arose out of struggles and controversies. They are based on irreconcilable polarities and ultimately will be destroyed by them, even if everybody ate only fruit and walked around naked. Even if my teachings about a healthy lifestyle were to gain a significant popularity, the general resistance to the change would cause a very slow transformational process in the economy of supply and demand resulting in a harmonious self-regulating, adaptation. The idea of paradise for the whole of humanity will remain utopian. Only very few people will have the opportunity and the good fortune to frolic under the shade of fruit trees and live from the sustenance they provide. Ignorance, lack of discipline, lack of faith will drive most people into the camp of the opponents of my teachings for a very long time to come.

The collective question is not the topic of this book. We are dealing with the illness of the individual human being, not the illness which has befallen humanity.

But here and there a suffering person will experience a revelation after reading this book. Most likely the sufferer will have already gone through a plethora of allopathic, homeopathic and naturopathic remedies and treatments.

In a best case scenario the patient will have switched from alcohol to milk and mineral water, from meat to eggs and oatmeal and is quite disappointed about the persistence of the illness in spite of sticking to his new diet.

The sufferer will be left with an all-pervasive skepticism which will extend to the simple, clear and self-evident truths I advocate. 'Could all conventional medicine be nonsense? A horrifying idea. First I ate myself sick and now I am supposed to get healthy by eating only fresh fruit, raw vegetables and nuts? All the money I made and spent on conventionally packaged processed foods, on dinners with steak and lobster in fine restaurants, is supposed to not only have been a waste, but the cause of my illness?'

The testimonials of many healings will not convince many sufferers. I could supply a whole train car filled with such testimonials yet most sufferers will remain prisoners of their ingrained habits. Some people will eat fruit for a week and feel weak and miserable, then return to their prior food habits and condemn my teaching based on their one week experience.

But there will be a few who understand the true meaning of my teachings in its essence and who will muster the energy and discipline to live the Ehret way. These individuals will not be disappointed. They will live the results of my promise. They will move through the transformation from being a sick person to a genuinely vital, eternally "HEALTHY PERSON".

VI
Explanation of Photographs

Photograph 1. Taken during my military duty as a one-year volunteer. Despite my healthful appearance I was dismissed during my eleventh month because of neurasthenia and a weak heart. After my recuperation I never again experienced any heart problems during my adult life.

Photograph 2. Taken during my late twenties. It shows very clearly the strain and stress, the mindless and uninspired facial expression of a glutton and beer-drinker,who still considers his condition "normal".

Photograph 3. Taken before I fell ill. Already a considerable weight loss is observable.

Photograph 4. During my illness: chronic nephritis; father and brother had died from lung-diseases; mother had died from kidney complications. I had gone through two years of allopathic treatment without results. I was close to death. My age is usually estimated fifteen years above my actual age.

Photograph 5. After a few years practicing naturopathic healing methods and vegetarianism my state of health had significantly improved, but I was not yet fully healed. At the time of the picture I had returned to eating raw and cooked food, but I already had started my fasting cures. This photograph was taken two days after fasting for thirty-two days.

Photograph 6. Four days after my fasting experiment, having eaten fruit only for two days and feeling already extraordinarily strong, in good spirits and agile. At the beginning of my illness I had experienced considerable loss of hair and graying. The photograph shows how my fasting cures regenerated the growth of hair.

Photographs 7 and 8. New pictures after my completed regeneration.

VII
Testimonials About Arnold Ehret's
Way to Health

Documentation and Healing Results

Article from the Journal "Lebenskunst" *(The Art of Life)*
Year 1912, Issue 9

Should We Take the Healing Diet of Arnold Ehret
from Locarno Seriously?
Author: Paul Liberner, Munich.

Every age has specific dietary recommendation for
its patients. Our times are made fascinating by a plethora of
voluntary and involuntary fasting cures, attributing to them
not only the panacea for gluttony, but also salvation from
every other burden afflicting the body or mind. Some medical doctors, who are normally scientifically oriented, have
already begun recommending fasting to their patients as an
inexpensive, yet effective way to health.

The master of this new movement is Arnold Ehret
from Locarno. It would be blasphemous to label this movement heresy, because all real saints of the Catholic Church
did extensive fasting.

Of course, physical self-castigation and abstinence
from food as well as hunger-artists who want to fatten their
purse through fasting demonstrations have been around for

quite some time.

But the former professor and painter Arnold Ehret has elevated the art of fasting into the dimension of the scientific experiment conducted in the laboratory of his own body. He has brought structure and purpose to this healing art which, generally speaking, is simple and yet profound in its potential for both radical healing and dangerous consequences. In repeated fasting experiments Arnold Ehret has proven to a large public the validity of this "ultimate healing method". He fasted in a glasshouse sealed by a notary for 49 days in the city of Cologne. To the many readers of his book "The Cause and Cure of All Illness" this unique experimenter describes his own healing process which transformed him from a deathly ill person to a completely healed individual through systematic fasting and proper nutrition (predominantly fruit).

Ehret soon became a well-known and much sought after speaker who gathered a large following of friends and fans around there. His fans demanded the living word of their leader and Ehret responded with workshops and a lecture tour through Germany after a similar, very successful tour through Switzerland last year.

His first stop was Munich, right in the middle of the Salvator-Strongbeer season, which coincides with lent. Ehret's first "fasting sermon" carried the title "The Cure for the Unhealed". The people of Munich came in large crowds, temporarily switching from the imbibing of Salvator-Strongbeer to the salvation-from-illness speeches of fasting apostle Arnold Ehret. They also came to his second lecture: "Are All Diseases Curable?" and they signed up for the workshops during the following three weeks.

Munich, the beer capitol of the world, had never before seen such an event, this diversion of the masses from 'beeretism' to 'Ehretism'. The public was more than idly curious. Their interest was genuine, their longing for a message with true value filled an essential human need.

The public lectures were full of useful information, which were reviewed extensively by the local newspapers. The more intimate workshops turned out to be invaluable sources of eternal wisdom.

Ehret solves the most simple and the most complex issues of living a healthy life with brilliantly convincing eloquence. He is an outstanding original orator, convincing to others because he himself is so convinced of his teachings. He looks radiantly healthy, and fascinates his audience from the first to the last word. In all his lectures Ehret aims at one cardinal truth: "The genuinely healthy person is capable of experiencing everything in its true beauty and magnificence. Become truly healthy." In spite of weeks filled with lectures, the audience never grew tired. The "suffering" ill person and the "healthy" person were portrayed from ever new perspectives and his disciples and listeners understood increasingly that Ehret, the great master of fasting, was backed up by eternal, undeniable truth.

Every session was followed by a question and answer period. Ehret provided answers for even the most difficult questions and amazed his audience with an original, precise and indisputable logic. Some questions led to somewhat embarrassing and inconvenient answers—for the questioner.

There were medical doctors among the audience. Although they could not officially agree with him, they quietly recognized his work and his empirical experiments, which were conducted on his own body.

It would be desirable for Ehret's critics to attend some of his workshops. He would cure their skepticism or at least modify it. Ehret is not the "mucus-fanatic" as he is sometimes portrayed. He certainly does distinguish between the formation of necessary mucus and pathological mucus. He does not claim mucus to be the only cause of every disease, but he sees it as the main cause, which is present in almost all diseases. Ehret also does not see himself as the exclusive "emperor" of fasting. He only claims to have brought system, structure and purpose to this ancient healing method, thereby elevating it to a legitimate healing method for our times. The gratefulness and appreciation of many former sufferers from severe illnesses confirms his choice of an effective method.

Maybe Ehret could be called "biased", but only by someone who has not studied his theories and practice. In diagnostic or therapeutic procedure Ehret focuses much less on the name of the disease than on the condition of the sufferer. Do we not have to agree with him? Is it not true that a runny nose or a sinus infection can kill a person, if the whole body's immune system is weak? And is it not also true that the most serious diseases are conquered with ease by a strong, vital general condition?

Do we not have to admit that advocating fasting as the therapy of therapies works and should be used first before the various remedies of naturopathic medicine are administered. Ehret is not against natural methods of healing. We do not know yet whether Ehret is only aiming at physiological health or whether he has higher spiritual goals. We will find out more about his views on the subject in his forthcoming book "About the Healthy Human Being".

Meanwhile, Ehret's followers listen to him with a critical mind. In Munich his following grew by hundreds of people and is expected to grow further in Nürnberg, Leipzig, and Dresden.

Ehret's art is hidden between the lines of his books and cannot be reduced to "one diet fits all and solves all problems". The ill person stands at the center of his own healing process and an individualized approach is essential. Self-treatment should proceed with caution. Ehret is the last person to replace a physician who is trained in supervising fasting.

Ehret needs to be taken seriously. After our experiences in Munich we have to agree with Dr. Katz in Stuttgart who evaluates his work: "Such healing successes challenge the methods of modern medicine to the core and the allopathic approach will have to change if it does not want to lose much ground with the public".

A few verses given to the parting Ehret in Munich show the depth and heartful connection between teacher and disciples.

Thank you, beloved guest
You were more than words to us
You brought us life
So life can give more life.
Let us proclaim forever
To rise with Ehret's teachings
Above the demons of greed

Towards the nectar of the Gods
We greet you, our most beloved teacher
And part with you today.
Soon without toxins, mucus, plague and goo
We will rejoin you healed
According to your wise words and teachings.

Relevant Articles in Newspapers

A daily paper in Brussels, Belgium reports on March 27, 1907

The inexpensive life. Doctor Bullisson from Toledo (USA) has solved the difficult problem of living inexpensively in a most elegant and comprehensive manner. He lives mostly on air. He has found out that food intake and sleep are mostly addictions and he is doing almost completely without them now for thirty years. He eats only once a day and then only fruit and vegetables, but he considers even this habit excessive and balances its negative effects by frequent extended fasting periods. His last fasting cure stretched over seven weeks. He began on January 5, 1907 and only imbibed a little water and plenty of fresh air.

Dr Bullisson asserts that a person has eaten enough by the age of 15 to live off his own accumulated substance for another 85 years. Hunger is a disease which we have caused through bad habits. Sleep is another disease or rather a device of nature to protect us from gluttony. Dr. Bullisson proves his theories by resting only one hour per day while still noticing people entering and leaving his room. When he gets up papers spread around his bed show that he even writes during his resting period.

A picture in the "Chicago Examiner" portrays him in a long beard and a robe playing with his children around a snowman. He is robust, strong and healthy, takes long hikes and declares feeling rejuvenated after every fasting period like a twenty year old man. Inside his home he wears no clothes and requires his family members to follow the laws of nature the way he does. Mrs. Bullisson hesitated but finally joined in the lifestyle of her husband.

The "Tagesanzeiger" *(Daily News)* of Zurich reports on April 6, 1910

Upton Sinclair's Hunger Cure

Upton Sinclair, the well known American author who had reached instant fame with his novel "The Jungle" exposing the scandalous conditions in the American meat factories, now surprises the world with another sensational discovery. He has discovered the secret how to get and stay healthy. Sinclair had suffered for years from headaches, infections and other illnesses. Then he went on an intensive search for health. "I made all the mistakes a human being can make and tried all new and old remedies which were recommended or prescribed for me." Then coincidence brought him together with a lady who was bedridden for decades. He suffered from rheumatism, stomach problems, neurasthenia and depression, but now looked so healthy, so vital, so joyful, to the amazement of everyone. She revealed her secret to Sinclair. Fasting, fasting, extended fasting is the way to health. He describes in detail the phases of his healing. "On the first day, I was very hungry. My hunger felt violent and impatient. On the second morning I still was a little bit hungry, but then the hunger pains disappeared completely and my worries about food also left as if I had never eaten. Before my fasting period I always suffered from headaches. They continued only for the first day of my fasting and then they disappeared, never to return. On the second day I felt somewhat weak and laid down in the sun reading the whole day. I did the same on the third and fourth day. A certain physical lassitude and tiredness stayed with me accompanied by a great mental clarity. On the fifth day I felt stronger and went for a walk, then I began to write. Nothing surprised me more than the agility of my mind. I wrote and read more than I ever dared to imagine."

Sinclair lost 15 pounds in the first four days, but then only two pounds in eight days. After twelve days he broke the fast by drinking orange juice only for two days and then building a transition to drinking milk. Since the fast he feels healthy and vital.

In the meantime Sinclair has written a book with the title: "The Art of Healing Yourself and Staying Healthy".

What is especially interesting is the increase of mental clarity after fasting. Sinclair himself was very surprised by this and one has to experience it to believe it.

TESTIMONIALS FROM PHYSICIANS

Dr. Katz, owner and director of the natural healing center Hohenwaldau in Degerpoch near Stuttgart is an authority in natural healing methods and has 20 years of experience in healing through diet and fasting.

Dr. Katz wrote an article in the journal "Die Sonne" (The Sun) of July 15, 1912, Nr. 14, P. 109-110.

Diet

The healing dietitian and diet reformer Arnold Ehret of Ascona spent July 2-8 in Stuttgart and gave his lectures as well as a course dealing with healing diets. He had a large and very attentive audience. Ehret's teachings link the well being or the illness of every individual to diet and maintain the mandatory imperative of a mucusless diet which consists of fruit and berries, vegetables, salad greens, soured milk, very little bread and a minimum or no cooked carbohydrates like noodle, pasta, etc. The mucusless diet is so crucial because Ehret sees the build up of mucus in the body and its organs as the first and foremost cause of disease. Health can only be achieved when this mucus is removed from the body. After much reflection and collection of empirical evidence with his patients Ehret came to the indisputable conclusion that his theory corresponds to the deeper truth of nature. Ehret healed many patients who had gone through many other therapies including very strict diets without results. After following his regime of a mucusless diet they all regained their health in a very short time.

Ehret also strongly advocates fasting and considers it the best and most successful curative therapy. Fasting is the method which all sick animals use instinctively until they regain their health. Fasting is the safest and never failing universal remedy, the foundation of all ways towards health.

The lecture was delivered with simplicity and humbleness, the arguments so cogent and compelling that his audience was convinced beyond doubt. The author of this letter thanked the speaker for his knowledge and asked the people present to follow Ehret's advice in practice. My own personal experience with patients verifies Ehret's teachings and I wholeheartedly recommend his way to health. Whoever wants to stay healthy or wants to regain his health will achieve his goal in the shortest possible time. Every doctor knows from experience that patients rarely like to change their diet and often hate restrictions. They rather cultivate their illness than follow the new dietary guidelines. Fasting is especially unpopular although it is not a difficult therapy when handled correctly. I recommend fasting under consistent medical supervision because of possible complications for the inexperienced practitioner.

Dr. Katz

The Cologne Experiment

Your triumph makes modern medicine obsolete and it will have to change its course and methods if it does not want to lose its role in society.

Dr. Katz

Stuttgart-Hohenwaldau, October 18, 1911

It is of paramount importance to educate the world about fasting and you are the most competent representative of fasting as a healing method.

Dr. Katz

Stuttgart- Hohenwaldau, August 14, 1911

Honorable Mr. Ehret

Thank you for giving me your book "Kranke Menschen". The content of your book brought me great joy and I totally agree with you. It is important to approach the subject cautiously because most people have a hostile attitude to your method, but it is the only solution, the only effective and safe way to health.

Dr. Katz

Stuttgart-Hohenwaldau, November 4, 1912

I believe we will convince the world that you are showing the right way and that without a true etiology a safe therapy is impossible.

Dr Katz

I think very highly of fasting as a curative method. In the next issue of the magazine "Die Hausarztin" (The General Practitioner) we will bring a longer article about your method.

Dr. Fischer-Dückelmann

A great interest in your subject causes me to see you. Your new insights based on empirical research conducted on your own body deserve everybody's attention. Your work is bringing clarity to many scientific questions.

Dr. K. in H.

Honorable Mr. Ehret!

I have read your letter (the teaching lesson concerning fasting and the mucusless diet) immediately with great excitement. After the third reading I slowly calmed down. Your method makes more sense than anything I have read! You really hit the nail on the head! My God! I asked myself: What am I studying medicine for? To become a surgeon? I am looking forward to meeting you soon;

> Respectfully
> N.H., medical student
> Freiburg i. Breisgau, March 6, 1909

The former drawing teacher in the secondary school in Freiburg i.B., Mr. Arnold Ehret as been known by me for a long time as a man who is fasting publicly not out of sensational or material motives, but out of a deep inner conviction and scientific interest in a healing method whose life saving effectiveness he has experienced on his own body.

If an educated person like Ehret demonstrates publicly the safety of long fasting periods for the human organism, it is not to impress spectators, but to promote a scientific and empirically proven most significant healing method. Mr. Ehret offers to all scientific observers a most conscientious and therefore truly valid conduct of his experiments.

> Dr. K. Bernold Martin

Mr. Arnold Ehret, born in 1866 in St. Georgen, told me today about his intention to conduct a fasting experiment here in Zürich. I have gathered information about his previous experiences in this matter and the specific details of the planned experiment. I have come to the conclusion that Mr. Ehret has the necessary knowledge and experience to conduct such an experiment.

I also believe that such an experiment conducted carefully without excess deserves the public attention and will have a positive effect on the public opinion.

Dr. M. Bircher-Benners Sanatorium
"Lebende Kraft (Lifeforce)
Zürich, Keltenstr. 8

I attest gladly, based on my experiences that it is possible to fast 50 days with 10 days of water intake, if someone has the training in this area. Your undertaking has a high scientific value from a medical as well as biological point of view.

Respectfully,
Dr. Mader, Sanatorium
Bad Gesundbrunn

I have known the secondary school teacher Arnold Ehret in Freiburg for eight years. I was his physician when he suffered from chronic kidney problems, neurasthenia and heart complications. It was a delight to be a witness to his healing. Mr. Ehret and other patients demonstrated the great value of methodically administered fasting cures which of course need to be adjusted to each individual case. There are no rigid rules here, but the creative art of healing through the guidance of an experienced physician.

It is in the public interest to witness the effects of genuine fasting in order to show the possibilities and the safety, the physiological changes of this method and therefore to alter our false notions about nutrition, illness and healing. I endorse the plans of my former patient to conduct public fasting demonstrations under strict supervision in various cities. Ehret is a man of absolute integrity and his enthusiasm for the cause of fasting guarantee the proper realization of such an undertaking.

Dr. G. Riedlin

I know several patients who completed an Ehret fasting cure. They ate nothing but a few apples and beets daily and lost considerable weight while staying in perfect condition. Such experiments are interesting because they show that civilized man eats much too much. It would behoove physicians to read Ehret's book on fasting and in spite of reservations I have I believe he points the way to possibilities for curing diseases valid for everyone. (Unfortunately his work also contains some misunderstandings.)

Prof. Dr. Carl L. Schleich
Berliner Tageblatt (Berlin Daily News),
Nr. 622, December 8, 1913

Testimonials from People Who Have
Put Theory into Practice

*Finally I would like to include a few testimonials
from people who understood my teachings, put them into
practice and who acknowledge and praise for the truth of
my work.*

—*Arnold Ehret*

Your two articles from the journal "Lebenskunst"
(The Art of Life) were a delight to read. It is strange what
intense seeking spreads through every human being even
though we are misled from a young age on.

It is beyond words to convey the impact your teachings had on me. My whole house, seven people, live according to your principles and we are blessed with healthy joy
and peace. Recently a friend full of mucus visited us and
was so impressed by my example and my explanations that
he adopted your principles immediately. This man, 31 years
old, was close to suicide and was transformed to a happy
human being. He is infinitely grateful. I feel like a new person myself and lost 42 pounds in one year.

I eat twice a day: at lunchtime and at dinnertime,
and almost exclusively mucusless food. You are a great
benefactor of mankind.

Thank you for your recent letter. Of course you can
quote me. I would be happy for all people if they lived
according to your principles and if I could contribute to the
spread of your message with my name, it would be to the
advantage of everyone.

My health is great. My emotional disposition outstanding, my voice gains in power and clarity as confirmed by my friends and the press. My body has more energy now than I have felt in 20 years. My whole physique has changed. I used to be puffy, fat and pale, but now I have a youthful figure and a healthy complexion. You can imagine what this means in my profession. I also have not been "nervous" for a year.

Every person can face his future without worries if he lives according to the laws of nature: simplicity and moderation.

Cordial greetings from your ever grateful
H. Knote, Royal Chamber Singer

I am happy to own the secret of fasting and the mucusless diet. Use my last letter if you want. I am delighted to support your cause. After my return I will contact you again and hope to serve you even more with the results of my service.

Berlin. W.9. Potsdamerstr. 6
E. Witte, Patent Lawyer

Your views differ from most others, but I believe you are right. I especially appreciate your attitude towards conventional medicine. You do not make the mistake of so many laymen in condemning it completely. You rather want to supply methods to prevent and heal diseases based on your practical experience.

Seb. Buchner, Engineer, Munich

Never, and I say that without exaggeration, have I seen the problem of the embodying spiritual energy treated with such authority and power.

> Major Lieutenant H. in H.

I am very interested in your work and will advocate it in every way. You do great service to science, much more than some highly decorated scholar who often sits on unearned laurels.

> With great respect and appreciation
> S., Principal in Sch.

After the publication of my book I feel I have a right to consider myself in the company of Metschnikoff (Professor in Paris, famous for his research on the causes of aging) and Ehret as the prophet of a new "physiological religion".

> Author P.A. in Vienna

Since you are not speaking in Nürnberg in the near future I would like to ask you for some information about "Ehretism".

Before I do that I would like to relate the deep gratitude of my wife and myself for being completely healed after following your cure. My wife suffered from a prolapsed uterus and was treated for several years without success by several doctors who declared her incurable. Not only did the condition disappear, but her whole body has achieved a vitality, flexibility and strength which I considered previously impossible. She works from 4:00 a.m. to 11:00 p.m. at home and in the business without help. It is impossible to list all the good things which came our way through your cure and we just thank you again and again for the great blessings you have brought to us.

Ehret's cure made us healthy but now we want to become full Ehretists. How can we do that?

Nürnberg, July 14, 1913

R. Klempt

My response comes from a spontaneous sense of gratitude after reading your article "The Experiment of a 49 Day Fast" in the journal "Vegetarische Warte" (Vegetarian Observer). I have been searching for eight years and gone through many stages of doubt, courage, joy of life and doubt again: who has the answer in the various vegetarian ways? What a joy it is to suddenly find someone who reads like the genuine truth. You start with radical assumptions and your evidence for the cause of all physical evil and the means of improvement first are shocking, but my quiet inner voice agrees with your radical analysis. Your reflections reached me just at the end of a 14 day fasting period. After reading your deliberations several times I feel strengthened in my conviction to continue on the path you propose and hope to return to Locarno someday.

Louise H. in Berlin

Vienna, January 22, 1911

Dear M. Ehret!

I just have to express my joy. I just finished your article: "Thus Speaketh the Disease" and can find only superlatives of my enthusiasm. I told a friend that your unique experiment, your conclusions in your previous articles about the true nature of disease are without exaggeration the greatest treasure ever found in the realm of health.

I wish there were more people who appreciated your actions and words. Continue your writing because you have too much to reveal.

Yours respectfully,
Gustav G. Steiner, Vienna I, Makartgasse 3

On Christmas Day of last year I lost my sight in both eyes through an infection which had occurred repeatedly in previous years and was treated without success. The eyelids were paralyzed and if opened by force, I could not distinguish between fingers of my hand in front of my eyes. General nausea and headaches kept me in bed since December 22. I called for Mr. Arnold Ehret (from Freiburg, Sandstr. 6) who had healed himself from a terminal disease. Following his recommendations I had immediate relief and noticed the return of my eyesight already on the 28th of December. All other symptoms subsided and today I have no problems with my eyes.

I owe the permanent cure of my eyesight to Mr. Ehret and I am willing to testify to this anytime in public.

St. Georgen i. Breisgau
June 30, 1907
Maria Rodiger

Other Ehret Literature Publishing Company Books

The Mucusless Diet Healing System by Arnold Ehret. A complete and workable program for cleansing, repairing, rebuilding and maintaining a healthy body.

Rational Fasting by Arnold Ehret. The book explains how to fast correctly and form lifetime dietary habits with the proper way of fasting. This message can last throughout your life.

The Grape Cure by Johanna Brandt. The author offers her personal contribution toward the solution of the Cancer problem and her personal experiences in trying to overcome this dreaded ailment. This book is intended more as a Cancer preventive.

Watch for the next Ehret book due out in 2002. It will be a translation of Ehret's personal hand written notes and his memoirs. The translation of his lecture notes from Ascona, Switzerland will follow.

The Ehret Literature Publishing Company, Inc.
P O Box 24
Dobbs Ferry, New York 10522-0024
www.arnoldehret.org